Praise for Menopause

"I really like your explanation of the body's systems. I also like the case histories your own personal additions about yourself. I am very impressed with the wide range of issues you address that are vital to our health and well-being. A really great book!"

— Lisa Smith, psychotherapist, Encinitas, CA

"I am simply overwhelmed about the way you have given so much information in such a delightful, warm manner. This book shows intense research, careful organization, many sources for data, and many persons of medical authority as a source for your comments. It is an incredible feat to combine comprehensive medical information in a charming, friendly style that does not overwhelm the readers. I am greatly impressed by your way of letting the reader view all the information and make her choice of treatments, techniques, and decisions. You don't have a dogmatic approach. You present sweeping research and authorities of real reliability, and then let the reader make her personal choice. In addition to all of this, your heart-appealing stories of your patients touches the reader's desire for a story element in the midst of all the medical information."

— Lois Shade, patient

"Terrific! Thank you, Dr. Carolle! There has been a need for someone to explain this in plain English for the layperson, with no medicalese. Your book helps us demystify our anatomy and our body . . . and it empowers us! Your personal stories read like an inspiring, motivational story of hope and triumph over adversity—they make me feel that anything—any dream—is possible, similar to the feeling I get when I'm with you personally. Thank you for the 'Our Bodies, Ourselves' for Menopause."

— Cheryl Geer, D.O., OB-GYN

"Dr. Jean-Murat provides solid information combined with good practical advice in an easy-to-follow format. She dissects the complex issues of menopause into easy-to-digest bite-size pieces. Recommended reading for all perimenopausal and menopausal women. . . ."

— Nancy Cetel, M.D., reproductive endocrinology-menopause specialist, Encinitas, CA

"In this remarkably readable and warmly personal book, Dr. Carolle combines solid scientific knowledge with a healthy respect for multiple approaches to healing. She treats the body as a whole, profoundly interconnected—body, mind, and spirit. The book is a great mixture of folk wisdom, personal testimonies, and medical expertise. It encourages women to accept the seasons and changes in their bodies as 'natural occurrences' rather than 'diseases that must be treated with drugs.' At the same time, she suggests remedies, medications, and surgical procedures if and when that treatment is indicated. This book is a 'must have' resource for every woman, of whatever age, who wants to stay alive as long as she lives."

— Beth Glick-Rieman, author of Peace Train to Beijing and Beyond

MENOPAUSE
MADE EASY

Also by Carolle Jean-Murat, M.D.

Natural Pregnancy A–Z

Staying Healthy: 10 Easy Steps for Women
(published in both English and Spanish)

Other Hay House Titles of Related Interest

Emerging Women: *The Widening Stream,*
by Julie Keene and Ione Jenson

Empowering Women: *Every Woman's Guide to Successful Living,*
by Louise L. Hay

Growing Older, Growing Better: *Daily Meditations for
Celebrating Aging,* by Amy E. Dean

The Love and Power Journal: *A Workbook for the Fine Art of Living,*
by Lynn V. Andrews

(All of the above titles are available at your local bookstore, or may be
ordered by calling Hay House at 800-654-5126.)

Please visit the Hay House Website at: **www.hayhouse.com**

MENOPAUSE MADE EASY

How to Make the Right Decisions for the Rest of Your Life

CAROLLE JEAN-MURAT, M.D.

Hay House, Inc.
Carlsbad, California • Sydney, Australia

Published and distributed in the United States by:
Hay House, Inc., P.O. Box 5100, Carlsbad, CA 92018-5100
(800) 654-5126 • (800) 650-5115 (fax)

Editorial supervision: Jill Kramer • *Book design:* Jenny Richards
Illustrations: Carolle Jean-Murat

Library of Congress Cataloging-in-Publication Data

Jean-Murat, Carolle.
    Menopause made easy   :   how to make the right decisions for the rest
of your life   /   Carolle Jean-Murat.
            p.   cm.
    Includes bibliographical references.
    ISBN 1-56170-606-X   (tradepaper)
    1. Menopause Popular works.   2. Middle aged women–Health and
hygiene.   I. Title.
RG186.J43   1999
618.1'75–dc21   99-21387
                                                                CIP

ISBN 1-56170-606-X

04 03 02 01   7 6 5 4
First printing, June 1999
4th printing, August 2001

Printed in Canada

*To my husband, Albert, who makes me feel up to any challenge.
To my family, my friends, my colleagues, and everyone who makes it
easy for me to care for my patients. To the memory of my paternal
grandmother (Grandma), Eugenie Jean; my maternal grandfather,
Mirabeau Murat; my friend Shirley Day Williams; my adopted Jewish
mother Hinda C. Larkey; and "Pappy" Necker Duvalsaint.*

To the women of the world without a voice.

Contents

PART II: LIFESTYLE CHANGES

PART III: FOR FURTHER REFERENCE

APPENDIX

FOREWORD

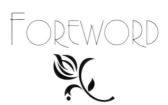

In 1998, the North American Menopause Society announced a new Gallup survey of 752 women ages 50 to 65 who had reached menopause. The survey revealed that 51 percent of the women said that they had "never felt as fulfilled and happy as now." This attitude is in stark contrast to the perspective portrayed just three short decades ago, when David Reuben, the author of *Everything You Always Wanted to Know About Sex,* wrote:

> Having outlived their ovaries, they may have outlived their usefulness as human beings. The remaining years may just be marking time until they follow their glands into oblivion.

Imagine! This was published in the late 1960s, albeit by a man. We certainly have come a long way, baby.

Another startling statistic is that every seven seconds a baby boomer turns 50. This amounts to 5,000 women per day, or 2 million per year. All in all, we can expect the already 40 million postmenopausal women to swell their ranks by some 20 million in the next decade. That's a lot of fulfilled and happy women! But what about health? We know that women are more likely to live longer than men, but often with more chronic disease and disability.

From a medical standpoint, we are still not certain of the best course to recommend to all women for relief of menopausal symptoms and prevention of long-term diseases. Because of the uncertainties and contradictions emerging from traditional medicine over the past decade, women are increasingly frustrated, and, accordingly, seek other options. The challenge, however, for women and health-care providers alike, is to recognize the strengths and shortcomings of the various options currently available. While more and more research is being done to address these questions, the answers are still another decade off, while women want to do something *right now!*

In *Menopause Made Easy,* Dr. Jean-Murat attempts to recognize the choices available and point out what we know, what we don't know, and the uncertainties of each. This is a formidable task, and one that she has risen to with her own very personal style. She writes the book as a physician and as a woman with her own experiences and philosophy woven into the tapestry of her message. Her rich personal history with alternative healing provides a strong foundation for her multidisciplinary approach.

For the woman trying to maneuver through her own menopause, this book should provide a free-thinking alternative to help navigate the changing terrain as the years of her menopause transition evolve. While we must constantly be aware of emerging data and new findings that may challenge our old ways of thinking, given what we know right now, *Menopause Made Easy* is a good place to start!

— Cynthia A. Stuenkel, M.D.
Associate Clinical Professor of Medicine,
University of California, San Diego

PREFACE

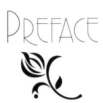

"I don't want to just practice medicine—
I want to LIVE it. It's in my blood. . . ."
— Carolle Jean-Murat, M.D.

I was born in Port-au-Prince, the capital of Haiti, in 1950, the first-born daughter of Joseph Karl Jean, and Marie Anne Lamercie Murat. My mother's father was Mirabeau Murat, one of the best known Voodoo priests and indigenous healers in Bizoton, a small town outside of Port-au-Prince. No one in my mother's family had ever graduated from primary school. In contrast, my father came from a family where being a lawyer, judge, or teacher was the norm. My paternal grandfather was a pharmacist and an alcoholic. Due to his abusive behavior, my father left home as a teenager to fend for himself.

I was four years old and my sister Marise had just turned two when my father left my mother. Distraught, my mother took us to my paternal grand-mother's home—not just for a visit—but to stay forever. Because of my mother's dire financial straits, we had to be "given" to Grandma and my Aunt Julia, my father's sister who had never married. We called her Tatante. She was adamant that Marise and I be raised without any ties to my moth-er's family.

After a painful parting, the occasional visits to my mother were so upsetting that I promised her that someday I would become important and take care of her so she would never have to cry again. When I made the decision that I would never to be caught in the same educational, economical, and socially dependent position as my mother, I was ten years old.

I grew up in an oppressed political milieu, in a country with very little resources, where political strife was common. I was six years old when Papa Doc Duvalier came into power, and his son Baby Doc and I are the same age. I lived through the political repression of a dictatorship. People were being killed at will in the name of "eradicating communism." Neighbors and friends just "disappeared." One of my uncles, Tonton Charlemagne, went to get some fresh air while waiting for my Aunt Antonine to prepare supper, and never returned. To this day, his clothes are still in the closet waiting for him.

Schools would close at the first sign of political unrest. However, Tatante made sure that I studied at home, and she helped me with my homework. She also hired a private tutor for me so that I could pass the National Exam to enter secondary school. I did not have any girlfriends because I was mostly interested in being a tomboy, and in reading. I would stay up reading even though there was a blackout every night for several hours. Grandma always worried that I was going to lose my sight reading so many hours by candlelight.

Books were rare to find. They were considered communist propaganda by the Duvalier regime and had been banned or burned. Fortunately, a friend of the family, Clovis, had a large, secret library at his home. One day when I was a teenager, I asked him to lend me one of his books to help with my homework. He did, reluctantly. The cover of the book was somewhat torn, so with great care I repaired it. It looked like new when I returned it. Clovis was so impressed that he said I could borrow as many books as I wanted. I was elated!

Thanks to Clovis, I learned so much from many wonderful books. I was most influenced by a quote from Montaigne: "Women are not in the wrong when they decline to accept the rules laid down for them, since the men made these rules without consulting them. No wonder intrigue and strife abound." I also liked reading about George Sand, a woman writer who dressed like a man and smoked a cigar!

When I read *The Second Sex* by Simone de Beauvoir, I was very impressed that she dared to be different. She asked why women did not dispute male sovereignty, and why a category of people dominated another. But she noted that it was not always the case, giving the Negroes of Haiti as an example. I grew proud of my Haitian heritage. The Haitian slaves, against all odds, had defeated "invincible" Napoleon's army.

I was going to be different, too, I promised myself. I was not going to be like the many girls I knew who only wanted to be married, have kids, and be subordinate to their men. I was going to be smart and go as far as any man could ever go.

I was going to be a champion of hope!

❧ ❧ ❧

I lived in a caste society in Haiti, but I was fortunate that my paternal grandfather's station in life established us in Port-au-Prince. The people of Lacou Mirabeau, on my mother's side, were "low-class and evil," according to my parochial school and the society I lived in. And so, I was challenged by being raised to deny the merits of my mother and her family. My mother's family, whenever I could see them, would shower me with love and the hope that I would make a better world for them because of the opportunities that I had in Port-au-Prince.

The societal class system was so strong that the prestigious Catholic school that I was attending kicked me out when they learned about my maternal origins. My maternal grandfather, Mirabeau, the well-known indigenous healer, was considered to be from a "low class." The impact of this discrimination caused me to become very ill. Grandma took me to the established doctors who were unsuccessful in improving my health. My mother, upon learning I was not well, insisted on taking me to my grandfather. His healing ability restored my health, which made a great impression on me.

Having to live in a society that consistently denied a part of me only increased my determination to succeed. During my occasional visits to Grandfather Mirabeau, he reassured me that I would be a healer like him, but that because of my paternal family's influence, I would acquire the skills I needed in formal medical school. He promised me that he would be available for "second opinions."

Under such severe conditions and with mixed emotions, how was I able to remain strong? In spite of my aunt's prejudiced attitude, my father and grandma were my unwavering supports. My father worked for the government and in other odd jobs all over Haiti. This made his visits very infrequent and our relationship more endearing, even though I was also torn with resentment over the fact that he had left my mother.

Sometimes for months at a time, my father would not receive a paycheck from the government. Even though my grandma could find some work as a seamstress, and Tatante also helped, we went through hard times. We could have had an easier life if my father had joined the *tontons macoutes*, Papa Doc's secret service, but Father was against bearing arms. I remember lying in bed at night with an empty stomach, unable to sleep. Grandma would sit by my bedside and rub my belly and pray with me: *"Une mauvaise nuit bientot passee"* (a bad night should soon come to an end). After she left, while I tossed and turned in the dark, I never thought of going to the pantry to eat what she had set aside for the next few days. Grandma was adamant that "we do not eat the turkey today and the feathers tomorrow." We had to learn to live on what we were allocated for that day.

Whenever he visited us, my father would reiterate that as his children, we could pursue whatever we wanted to be, erasing any doubts I had about being a trailblazer. At each visit, Father would have me rub the palms of his hands, which were covered with calluses due to hard labor, to remind me of how hard he was working to support all my dreams. I was a lucky girl, since at that time, higher education was reserved for boys. Because of my father, I grew up believing that there was nothing I could not do. When tough situations would arise, I was not allowed to doubt my ability or to put my dreams to rest.

To me, Grandma was a daily role model and a constant reminder to be humble. Even though she barely knew how to read and write and did not know of any woman doctors, she believed that *I* could be one. She always talked about Albert Schweitzer's hospital, where the poor could receive free medical care. Sometimes they would have to walk for days to get there. Grandma also shared the stories of her childhood and how she endured life in a man's world. As an ingenious and industrious woman who found loopholes in the court system to remedy the injustices imposed on Haitian women who had no rights, she feared nothing—not even the devil!

Grandma had a special bag that contained many smaller ones, each filled with different herbs. She knew all the herbs by name, and just how much to give you to make you feel better. She also practiced preventive medicine. Every six months or so, Grandma would disappear for a whole day. I found out years later that she was going all the way to the town of Leoganne, a small town south of Port-au-Prince, to see Madame Jean, a folk healer. She first had to take a taxi, then a special bus. The trip would last about two hours. Madame Jean was Grandma's "primary care" doctor.

One day, Grandma told me about her visits to Madame Jean. "When I get there, she gives me a large pot of some kind of mixture that I sip during my stay. She would then have me take off all my clothes, rub my whole body with special herbs, and give me some more potion to take with me." With this and her prayers, Grandma felt that she had nothing to fear as far as her health was concerned. Grandma was right as usual—she outlived Madame Jean and all her medical doctors.

Unfortunately, both my paternal grandfather and Grandma had already died when I became interested in alternative healing. I had lost the chance to learn from them forever.

Being in Grandma's care and having experienced firsthand my maternal grandfather's skills as an indigenous healer, I grew up with the understanding that healing had spiritual, mental, and physical components.

My very first experience as a future healer occurred while visiting my mother at age 11. That night, a neighbor requested my mother's help with an expected birth. I was unaware that my mother was also a healer. I begged to go along, stressing that I was a future doctor, making myself useful by carrying the small burner to light the way to the woman's house. We arrived just as the baby was on its way. I watched my mother calmly put everything in order and bring a new life into this world. I was affected by the whole event, and as I walked back, my thought was that I wanted to be a doctor, but I surely had to find a way to deal with all that blood!

❦ ❦ ❦

When I was 15 years old, my father came home one night all beat up to tell us that he had to leave in exile. A few days earlier, he had been snatched from home, handcuffed, tortured, and taken to Fort-Dimanche, an infamous prison, to be killed and thrown into an open grave. He was spared only because a childhood friend, a high-ranking *tonton macoute,* was present. But he got the message that they were going to be back, and this time he would not escape his fate. Fortunately, unlike the Haitians who had to leave by boat years later, my father flew to Martinique, and later to New York, where he obtained immigrant status. Working two jobs, he was able to save money and apply for Marise and my sister Elsie to come to the United States, the land of opportunity.

What assured that I would be a healer and take care of the poor occurred to me when I was 16. My stepfather, Achilles, was the regional director for CARE, and one summer, I had gone to spend three weeks in a small town where a bridge had to be fixed. The workers would be paid with bags of powdered milk, wheat, flour, and oil. My stepfather was one of the few who made sure that the food was given to the poor.

Next to where we stayed was a small clinic, and the male nurse, Joseph, was there one day a week. I asked if I could help him. People would arrive from far away before the doors were opened. The clinic had acquired medications and supplies, donated by a religious group from the United States. Joseph listened with patience to all the complaints. For payment, Joseph would get a live chicken, a bag of fruits, eggs, or a little change. I learned that the people believed in injections, and the more they hurt, the better! When I noticed that some patients got only painful injections of sterile water and asked Joseph about this, he said that there was not enough medication to go around, and his only alternative was to give them the painful sterile-water injection. Most of these trusting people would be cured just by the fact that Joseph told them he was administering medication to heal them!

That experience confirmed my decision to be a doctor. The plan became: Complete pre-med in Haiti, go to the United States to join my father, and then proceed to medical school at a French-speaking university in Europe. When I left Haiti for the United States at the age of 20, I had big dreams. To my disappointment, I soon realized that the streets of America were not paved with gold! Not only that, prejudice reared its ugly head. My father had been adamant that education was a must. His daughters were to have an education and not be called disparaging names.

But I got accepted at the Autonomous University of Guadalajara, in Mexico, with an old classmate, Nicole, who shared my dreams and provided me lots of moral support. I spoke French, the official language of Haiti, as well as Haitian. I had to improve my Spanish skills, and since my goal was to be accepted into a postgraduate program in the United States, this meant that I also had to buy my medical books in English.

Money was scarce, but I was able to get ahead by implementing those survival techniques that I had learned from Grandma. I started to learn Italian and found a part-time job at the university translating scientific papers from Italian, English, and French into Spanish. When time permitted, I would type other students' papers, or give French lessons here and there to supplement the money my father sent.

Luckily I was able to find an internship in Jamaica with the University of the West Indies. Interns were paid up to $800 a month, with free room and board. There I was able to see many diseases and surgical cases that most students only read about, and I learned about labor and delivery from nurse midwives. It was hard work, but it was mitigated by the hospitality of the Jamaican people, such as Rita Robotham Moodie and her mother, Olive McKenzie; the wonderful Reggae music; and the excellent food.

During my year of community service in Mexico following my internship in Jamaica, I learned how to practice medicine in small towns and deliver babies on farms after riding there on tractors at night with a flashlight.

I had been writing to many hospitals in the United States inquiring about a residency, to no avail. Fortunately, because of a friend that I had met in medical school, I was accepted into a residency program in obstetrics and gynecology at Mount Sinai Medical Center, in Milwaukee, Wisconsin. I also had the opportunity to spend two months at the University of Madison for a rotation in the Department of Reproductive and Endocrinology Medicine, a major base of infertility and research in the Midwest and the University of California Los Angeles (UCLA), its counterpart on the West Coast.

My greatest challenge as a fledgling doctor came about when I arrived in Milwaukee. Being an intern meant having no more status than a pile of dirt! When on call, I was expected to be in three places at the same time: the labor and delivery ward, the emergency room, and the floors doing admissions. I also had to get used to the coldest weather of my life!

But the rigors of winter and residency training were offset by the hospitality and love of Jay Larkey, M.D., the head of obstetrics; his wife, Hinda; their daughters, Cindy and Debbie; and their son, Hirsh. They became my adopted Jewish family. Hinda reminded me of Grandma.

When I got to Mount Sinai in 1978, I had my share of dealing with people from all walks of life, races, and classes. My grandma had taught me to respect everyone I came in contact with, regardless of whom they were. "We are all the same," she used to say, "having to deal with life's circumstances." She also told me that I had the right to expect to be treated likewise. But I was appalled at the attitude of some of the doctors I had to work with. They were sexist, prejudiced, opinionated, and in some cases, blatantly racist. Female medical students, residents, and patients were treated as second-class citizens. There were 23 male surgeons, each one thinking that "his" way was the "only" way. You could never please them all.

I knew that it was a four-year commitment, but there was no way I was going to last under these circumstances. So I developed a strategy: I was going to do what was expected of me as their slave, use a cue card for each one, describing their likes and dislikes, then take them aside, one by one, for a heart-to-heart talk. My spiel was as follows: "This is a teaching hospital. If you are so good, why don't you teach me everything there is to know? I am here for four years, and I am not leaving until I am done. I am a woman who has great things to accomplish in her life. Why don't you be part of my greatness, and I will always remember you in a positive way?" It worked. I got through it, and then treated myself to a move to San Diego, California, to set up my practice in 1982. It was one of the most challenging times in my life, but the love and caring of William and Phyllis Zuidema, my adopted California parents, made it easier.

For 13 years, I was the only black female obstetrician-gynecologist (OB-GYN) in San Diego County. At that time, being a female was more of a liability than it is now. Originally there was a San Diego Women Physicians Association that catered to women physicians and female medical students. I became president. The association eventually folded ten years later when being a female physician actually became an asset to female patients!

Grossmont Hospital had never had a woman surgeon when I joined the staff, and I remained the only female surgeon for four years.

As an obstetrician and gynecologist, I felt that I could have the best of two worlds. I could do preventive medicine, and at the same time, perform surgery. I found out that I did not have the heart to deal with chronically sick and dying patients. What I wanted to do was educate women to take care of themselves.

In the beginning of my career, when I was not very busy, I could take the time to practice all that I had learned over the years. Soon, I became known as the doctor who had a holistic approach to caring for patients, who believed that a patient had the right to accept or refuse care. I was willing to work with patients who elected to go with alternative medicine techniques. I refused to have a busy practice that would not give me enough time to really listen to my patients. I felt that I was obligated to tell patients what the books said, but at the same time, I could be supportive of alternative care and healing practices.

Practicing medicine is often like using a sixth sense, where clinical knowledge *plus* what is happening to that particular patient help me make the right decision. Making the "right" decision can be extremely difficult, because the medical system is not always set up to support what is best for the patient. That was one of the many reasons that I decided to stop practicing obstetrics after ten years in private practice.

When I think about it, few doctors have had my diverse experience when it comes to healing. I have personally been very ill and cured by my grandfather, a traditional healer with primitive diagnostic methods. I have also been in touch with people from different backgrounds who view illness and death as being caused by natural or supernatural forces. These people do not believe in the healing power of pills, but believe that leaves and other natural objects have mystical powers. Others associate the healing process with touch and prayer.

I grew up in a society where many of the sick used home remedies first. If home remedies did not work, they would go to an indigenous healer or a voodoo priest. Seeing a medical doctor was a last resort. Treatment was usually a combination of conventional medical treatment and cultural healing, accompanied by the removal of a hex or spell. Hospitals were considered places where people went to die!

Back then, there were so many rituals when it came to taking care of the sick. The most intriguing ones were the postpartum rituals: For the first 40 days following a baby's birth, the mother could have no sexual encounters. She stayed home the first three days and couldn't take a shower or eat anything cold. If she had to go out, she would have to be back as soon as the sun went down. So different from the speedy "drive-through" deliveries of today!

I soon realized that Grandma was right: As human beings, we are all the same; we all welcome compassion and caring. These two gifts, when generously given, go a long way toward our recovery. Now, as a doctor myself, I use the most advanced tools, such as highly sensitive blood tests and high-tech scanners that can detect extremely small tumors in any part of the body. It is true that tests, medications, and surgeries are, in many cases, necessary. But many times, I have asked myself which of the elements of "medicine" are most important.

I have learned that as a healer, I have to treat the whole person, not just the breast or the uterus. When a patient is in pain, holding a hand or using a wet cloth to cool off the sweaty forehead of a woman in labor really works wonders.

I have learned that caring is the real healing power!

❧ ❧ ❧

My private practice is small, but I love it because I have time to treat my patients like people instead of numbers. I have patients who pay me out-of-pocket because they do not like how they are treated within the depersonalized, managed-care system. Paperwork pollutes my soul and takes time and energy from the women I want to help.

In 1987, after Baby Doc left in exile, I went back to Haiti to start a clinic for the poor. But it was bad timing. Eventually I want to practice medicine for free in Haiti.

What sustains me, besides being married to my soulmate, Albert, are patients who let me know from time to time the difference I have made in their lives.

I wrote this book for them, and for all women who wish to be empowered by medical truths and the natural facts of life—before, during, and after menopause.

ACKNOWLEDGMENTS

Many people helped with this labor of love.

Linda Meyers was the first person I brainstormed with about writing the definitive book on menopause. Leslie Joyce had the first pass at my writing, ably mending my "English as a fourth language." Laurie Gill, my walking partner, helped me stay focused and to change medical terms into reader-friendly prose. Karen Wilkening edited and refined the manuscript and kept asking, "Where is the EASY part of this menopause book?" until the various charts started to make sense.

I was blessed to have my soulmate, Albert, at my side. He never complained about all the time I spent away from him doing research, working on the computer and the phone, or reviewing a handful of papers on the way to a party. My sisters Marise and Elsie (both nurses); Maria, the child-care specialist; my brothers Leslie, the pharmacist; and Jacky, a future dentist, all live in the United States and assisted with Haitian research regarding menopause.

I was also helped and encouraged by my mother, Marie Anne Lamercie Murat; my father, Joseph Karl Jean; my aunts Julia Jean (Tatante), Audencie Murat, and Marie Anne Nerette; Gabriel Mathieu; Andre Aladin; Jean Charles Mathieu; my stepmother, Clarisse Petrus (Eka); my childhood friend Claude Labissiere St. Surin; and my dear sister-friend and medical school housemate, Nicole Cadet Alerte, M.D.

Special thanks to Alix Duvalsaint, the type of male friend and confidant that every woman should have! He read the manuscript to help me, and also to prepare for when his wife Edith goes through menopause.

Sirocoro Dumbia was my computer guardian angel, retrieving lost files and keeping my computer equipment—and my head—straight. My friend Edna Parish offered emotional support, as well as her great cooking.

Thanks also to my friend and therapist, Denise Giutsi-Bradford, who continues to help me understand myself and to solidify my dreams in the world of healing.

I would also like to thank the following people for their unwavering support given in ways that I can't even truly express: James Schaeffer, M.D., and his wife Ghislaine; Myron Schonbrun, M.D.; Alan Spector, M.D.; and Paul Pyka, D.O.; and their staffs.

I appreciate my friends in the medical field who reviewed the manuscript: fellow gynecologists Nancy Cetel, M.D.; Steve Brody, M.D.; Mihn Ho, M.D.; Alan Spector, M.D.; and Cheryl Geer, D.O.; along with doctors in other specialties: Iyabo Daramola, M.D., an internist and my soul daughter; and Robert L. Gillespie, M.D., a cardiologist.

Thanks, also, to the doctors in the lounges at Alvarado and Grossmont Hospitals who listened as the chapters were conceived and written, and who fed me ideas. I also received help from Akanke Celestin-Ramsey, R.N., N.P.; and Rebecca Charles, R.N. Friends and patients such as Sofia Shafquat; Florise Marie Etienne; Karen Gless, R.N., MFCC, Ph.D., sex therapist; Beth Glick-Rieman, the author of *Peace Train to Beijing and Beyond*; Lisa Smith, psychotherapist; Anassa Briggs-Graves; Cheryl Simon (Athea), my belly-dancing teacher; Dr. Bobbie J. Atkins; Kim Edstrom; Monique Theodore, R.N.; Henri Theodore, M.D.; Steven Van Camp, M.D.; Jerome Robinson, M.D.; Michael Keller, M.D.; Marwan Sabbagh, M.D.; Jennifer Logan, M.D.; Susan Foley, Ph.D., O.M.D, L.Ac. Acupuncture; Placide Francois, Ph.D.; Antonio Mathieu, Ph.D.; Sharon Courmousis; Dorothy Annette; Bonnie Meyer, R.N; Bernadette Francois, M.D.; Emily Gunther; Sue Varga and David Barnett of *Mind Grind*; my adopted twin A. Jean Pickus, R.N., M.S.N.; Dr. Doreen Borseth, a chiropractor; and Elaine Stevens of *Stevens Media Productions*—all gave me lots of feedback. Also, coach Sandra Schrift, due to her invaluable guidance.

When Louise L. Hay agreed to write a chapter for this book, I was inspired to reach even higher levels in my endeavor to educate and empower women. I am touched by her confidence in me. The staff at Hay House was also very helpful.

And, of course, a heartfelt thanks to my patients, who enthusiastically agreed to share their experiences.

❧ ❧

Introduction

Over the next two decades, some 40 million baby boomers will be passing through menopause. Like you, most of these women have been accustomed to being in control of their health and reproductive lives, but now find themselves bewildered by a variety of new and incomprehensible symptoms. Seeking more information, they attend seminars, read books, listen to tapes, join chat rooms on the Internet, and attend community support groups. Around them circles a vast array of conflicting tips and wisdom from the media, friends, and health-care providers. Most of these women are very confused. Should they start hormonal replacement therapy (HRT)? Or should they do nothing and "ride it out"? What about alternative holistic options?

Some cultures even lack a word for menopause: It is simply a time of change, often for the better. The childbirth years are over, and the passage may be rough, but eventually life returns to normal.

In 1992, the National Institutes of Health launched a $625-million, 15-year trial to study major disease conditions as they occur in women. Heart disease, stroke, osteoporosis, depression, and breast and colorectal cancer are major focal points of this ongoing study; but the influence of racial, cultural, and economic factors in the health of postmenopausal women is being examined as well. Termed the Women's Health Initiative, the trial involves 160,000 women ranging in age from 50 to 79, at 47 centers nationwide. It is a major breakthrough in women's health research, which to date has received far less funding and interest than research performed on and for men. For years, women's hormonal changes were considered to "skew" research results. But because the clinical data from this large and valuable study will not be available until 2005, women today must continue to educate themselves and choose wisely among the various options available to them for coping more comfortably with menopause.

How many times have you been given confusing guidance about menopause; the pros and cons of HRT; recommendations for nutritional supplements; and information on risk factors for breast cancer, cardiovascular disease, osteoporosis, and Alzheimer's disease? How often should you have a mammogram? If you've been on HRT for years, can you or should you stop? Are you increasing your odds for breast cancer by taking hormones? Are you truly decreasing your risk of heart disease by taking hormones? There are no easy answers.

The purpose of this book is to help you answer these questions and make the right decisions for *you*. By answering the questionnaires and using the charts provided, you can carefully weigh your personal risk factors for heart disease, osteoporosis, and breast cancer, while making the best choices for you.

This book also offers an opportunity to discover important things about your state of health and the habits that maintain your status quo. Changing habits can be very difficult—I can attest to that myself! Giving up dysfunctional behaviors and thought patterns requires the motivation to become *conscious* and *responsible* for your health, which may add up to a whole new lifestyle approach.

In this book, it is my great honor to include the wisdom of Louise L. Hay, the bestselling author of books such as *You Can Heal Your Life* and *Empowering Women.* Her positive philosophy and healing techniques have affected the lives of millions worldwide. In chapter 18 on "Healthy Aging," she explains how to accept and love our bodies, age gracefully, and rediscover our spirituality. I am blessed to have her in my life!

This book will supply you with extensive information about the female reproductive system; hormones (estrogen, progesterone, and testosterone); and their role in a woman's menstrual cycle and in her life generally. Perimenopause (the stage that precedes menopause) and menopause are covered in detail. Traditional and alternative treatments for perimenopausal and menopausal symptoms, including dosage risks and benefits, are also included.

This book also discusses diseases such as breast cancer, osteoporosis, cardiovascular disease, and Alzheimer's, all of which increasingly affect women as they age. You will learn how to moderate your risk of such diseases, receiving guidance for lifestyle changes that help to foster good health. You will also be given reminders to review your risks periodically as I help you "sage" (my term for aging with wisdom).

The goal of this book is to enable you to make educated choices by supplying you with the most pertinent information available. (Please check my website at **www.drcarolle.com** periodically for updated information and research results.)

There is a saying: Knowledge equals confidence, confidence is power; therefore, *knowledge is power*. May the knowledge you attain from this book empower you to consciously make the right decisions for the present stage of your life—and for all your years to come!

PART 1

Your Body and Your Health

CHAPTER 1

The Female Sexual and Reproductive Systems

To know what is really happening to your body you need to know how it really works. So let's review a little anatomy and biology. I'll try to make it as painless as possible!

Figure 1-a
THE VULVA

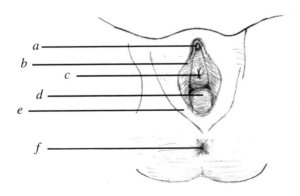

a) clitoris b) Labium minus c) urethral opening d) vaginal opening
e) Labium majus f) anus

Figure 1-b
INTERNAL ORGANS

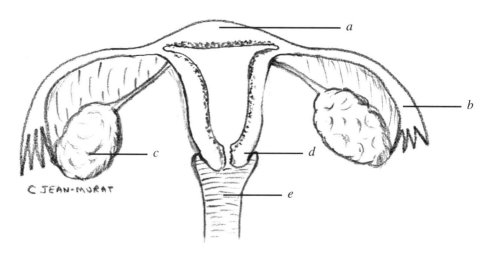

a) uterus   b) fallopian tube   c) ovary   d) cervix   e) vagina

Female Anatomy

The vulva: A woman's external genital area is called the vulva, or introitus.

The mons pubis: The mons pubis is a fatty prominence in front of the pubic bone that develops a layer of hair during puberty.

The labia minora: The labia minora, or inner lips, are two small folds situated between the labia majora (outer lips), originating at the clitoris.

The clitoris: The clitoris, a small bud-shaped organ, is the female equivalent of the male penis. It is located beneath a hood, a skin fold, extending to the superior end of the labia minora. The clitoris is generally a woman's most sensitive sexual organ.

The labia majora: The labia majora, or outer lips, are two prominent longitudinal folds, starting at the mons pubis and surrounding the clitoris, the labia minora, the urethra, and the vagina. They correspond to the scrotum in males.

The urethra: The urethra is a small, hollow tube that leads from the bladder, through which urine is excreted from the body. In the female, the urethral opening is situated below the base of the clitoris. In the male, it is also the passageway through the penis for the discharge of semen.

The mucosa of the vagina and the urethra are highly sensitive to the action of estrogen. Because of the proximity to the vaginal opening, some women are very prone to bladder infections. This is due to the introduction of bacteria during the sexual act.

Bartholin's glands: They are small glands located on either side of the vaginal opening that secrete a lubricating fluid during sexual arousal. In virgins, the vaginal opening is partly closed by the hymen, a delicate, elastic mucous membrane.

The vagina: The vagina is a three- to four-inch passageway extending from the uterus to the outside of the body. It functions as the female sexual organ and the birth canal.

The uterus: The uterus is an inverted, pear-shaped, hollow, muscular organ located in the female pelvic region between the bladder and the rectum. The wider body of the uterus is called the uterine fundus. The uterus provides the necessary environment for a fertilized egg to grow and mature into a baby. The uterus is covered by a smooth outer surface, the perimetrium. Its middle muscular layer is called the myometrium. The inner lining shed each month during menstruation is called the endometrium. In many cultures, the uterus is synonymous with sexuality, sensuality, and femininity.

The Fallopian tubes: On each side of the top of the uterus, coming out like a pair of arms, are the Fallopian tubes, through which the egg travels from the ovary to the uterus, and where fertilization occurs. Each tube is very mobile and measures approximately four inches long.

You may have heard of an "ectopic pregnancy." This is a situation where the pregnancy occurs outside of the womb. In most cases, it occurs in the Fallopian tubes.

The cervix: The cervix is the lowermost portion of the uterus, a narrow necklike end that opens into the vagina. This is the opening that dilates during childbirth. It is the site from which a Pap smear is taken. When a Pap smear is found to be abnormal, a colposcopy is performed. During the colposcopic exam, a speculum is inserted into the vagina, followed by a colposcope—a vaginal microscope that focuses an intense light, allowing for location of the abnormal cervical area. The health-care provider may take sample cells for examination. If necessary, cells can also be scraped from the cervical canal. The cervix varies in shape depending on whether or not a woman has had children. It can be palpated by inserting a finger into the vagina, and feels like the tip of the nose.

The ovaries: At the ends of the Fallopian tubes, on each side, are the ovaries—oval-shaped glands, the size of walnuts—containing multiple follicles (envelopes that hold an egg). At birth, a female child has approximately 450,000 follicles in her ovaries. They dwindle to about 50 by age 40.

During ovulation, one or two mature eggs is released. If the egg is not fertilized, it dissolves in the body. You've probably heard about fertility drugs such as clomiphene citrate, typically used to help infertile women ovulate. Usually, when a woman ovulates on her own, she has only one mature egg available for fertilization at a time. These drugs prompt many eggs to mature at the same time. They are generally used during natural intercourse, timed to coincide with ovulation, intrauterine insemination, or in vitro fertilization. Intrauterine insemination is when washed sperm are injected into the uterus at the time of ovulation. For in vitro fertilization, many eggs matured through fertility drugs are harvested and fertilized outside the womb. The fertilized embryos are then put back into the woman's uterine cavity. Multiple births may ensue.

The ovary is the site where the female sex hormones—estrogen and progesterone, and a small amount of the male hormone, testosterone—are produced.

Female Hormones—What They Do

Estrogen: Estrogen is responsible for bodily changes during adolescence—that is, the development of breasts and sex organs, the onset and regulation of the menstrual cycle, and reproduction itself.

Before puberty, estrogen is produced by the adrenal glands, which are located on top of each kidney. The ovaries take over at menarche (the onset of menstruation). The ovaries produce three types of estrogen; estradiol, estrone, and, to a lesser degree, estriol.

Once menarche begins, the principal circulating estrogen is estradiol. After menopause, when total estrogen production decreases by 70 to 80 percent, estrone becomes the predominant form of estrogen. Estriol, the weakest of the estrogens, is highest during pregnancy.

Estrogen is the dominant hormone present during the week that follows menstruation. It stimulates the buildup of the endometrium at the same time the follicle is growing within the ovary to develop an egg. Estrogen is also responsible for the changes occurring in the vaginal and cervical mucosa to make this environment more hospitable to sperm. Estrogen peaks at about 12 days after the start of menstruation, and then tapers off.

Estrogen is needed to maintain bladder and urethral mucosa, body muscles, skin tone, as well as to keep the vagina moist. Estrogen production continues after menopause. The amount of estrogen in the body after menopause depends upon body fat. In a study of obese women who were at least 20 percent over ideal body weight, estrogen levels were found to be 40 percent higher than in non-obese women. Estrogen is also derived from the conversion of androgens—the male hormones—in muscle, brain, skin, hair, and bone marrow.

Progesterone: Progesterone helps the lining of the uterus to thicken in preparation for a possible pregnancy. The main function of progesterone is to support pregnancy. Each month, during ovulation, the ovaries release one or two eggs into the Fallopian tubes, where they may be fertilized. After ovulation, progesterone is the predominant hormone. With the rise of progesterone, body temperature also rises about one degree Fahrenheit. After menopause, ovulation ceases, and there is no further production of progesterone.

Testosterone: The ovaries and adrenal glands produce a tiny amount of testosterone, the male hormone. Testosterone is involved in both the male and female sex drive (libido). It is also involved in bone and muscle growth and in sexual development. Testosterone is also produced by peripheral conversion of androgen precursors such as DHEA (dehydroepiandosterone) and androstenedione. At menopause, testosterone production drops by 50 percent.

Other hormones, such as insulin produced by the pancreas, and thyroid hormones, also affect menstrual cycles and bodily functions.

The Menstrual Cycle

Each month for 35 to 40 years between puberty and menopause, the female body prepares for the possibility of producing a baby. The reproductive system goes through a cycle of fertility that results in either menstruation or pregnancy.

Menarche, the onset of menstruation, occurs between the ages of 11 and 13 in most American females. At the beginning of the century, the average age of menarche was 14 to 15. A small number of girls begin to menstruate as early as age 9. It is speculated that menarche is triggered by a girl's weight and percentage of body fat, which in recent generations has been achieved earlier due to better health and nutrition. Some speculate that estrogen-like pollutants now being discovered in the environment may contribute to the early onset of menarche.

The average length of the menstrual cycle is 28 days, with a range of 23 to 39 days. The average blood loss is 40 milliliters (ml), with a range of 25 to 69 ml. Blood flow during the menses usually lasts for three days, with a range of two to seven days.

The pituitary gland is located at the base of the brain between the eyes. Another area of the brain is called the hypothalamus. Together they work to produce FSH (follicle-stimulating hormone) and LH (luteinizing hormone), which cause the ovaries to produce estrogen and the follicle to mature into an egg; and at midcycle, to trigger ovulation (the release of an egg).

The egg is caught by the Fallopian tube and carried into the uterus. Meanwhile, estrogen and progesterone prepare the lining of the uterus for the fertilized egg. If no fertilization occurs, the lining is shed, resulting in the menstrual flow. If intercourse has occurred, the egg may be fertilized by a sperm. Estrogen and progesterone also signal the pituitary to decrease FSH levels until the next cycle.

From day one to day five of the menstrual cycle, estrogen drops off, inducing a surge in FSH, which stimulates the follicle itself to produce estrogen and progesterone. From day 6 to day 14, estrogen rises and FSH falls. Days 14 to 28 bring an increase in estrogen and progesterone, followed by a fall.

This chapter should serve as a good foundation for the information that is to follow.

CHAPTER 2

Alternative Medicine

Alternative therapies are gaining increasing attention among patients and many health-care providers. In 1992, the National Institutes of Health established the Office of Alternative Medicine to fund research that includes studies of lifestyle changes; herbal remedies (including phytoestrogens, or plant estrogens); biofeedback; homeopathy; and acupuncture. In 1997, 83 million Americans spent $27 billion on chiropractic therapies, herbal remedies, and other alternative therapies. There were 386 million visits to primary-care physicians in 1997, compared to 629 million visits to alternative-medicine practitioners—a 50 percent increase from 1990.

This chapter is designed to give you some fundamental information about natural and alternative treatments for some of the symptoms of perimenopause and menopause. In addition, you will find a list of alternative practitioners at the end of this book.

To begin with, if you want to use alternative treatments, you need to be cautious, especially if you're taking prescription drugs. Herbs and food supplements may sometimes change the requirements for your prescribed medication. I recommend that you seek the help of a qualified practitioner.

Many women believe in "natural" approaches in order to avoid the side effects of standardized HRT. "Natural" means that the molecular structures are modified in the laboratory to match those found in the human body. Natural products may not necessarily be more effective or less toxic than their more traditional counterparts.[1] Furthermore, the production of so-called natural modalities may not be any more natural or less profit-driven than that of conventional hormones. Some companies falsely label their product "natural" because using the word helps sell products! Some alternative and conventional products are manufactured by the same multinational companies: profit-driven corporations with aggressive marketing plans.

In many cases, the health benefits of many products being marketed as "natural" have not been substantiated. Prescription drug formulations are regulated by the Food and Drug Administration (FDA), which tries to assure the safety and effectiveness of all drugs. The FDA also regulates the production, quality control, and advertising of every drug sold. Over-the-counter herbs and supplements lack quality control of content. There is usually a batch-to-batch variation. Quality control also varies between manufacturers, and there is a lack of human toxicological studies. Overall, this is a largely unregulated industry.

Consumers should be aware that they may be wasting their money. There is no law mandating that manufacturers of dietary supplements support their claims that their products actually help. In 1994, the Commission of Dietary Supplements recommended that natural claims be supported by scientifically valid evidence presented to the FDA, but this recommendation was quickly dropped. The FDA gets involved only when trouble is suspected, and it allows manufacturers to sell their products without any scientific proof.

Believe it or not, vitamins can be labeled "natural" with only 10 percent of the content actually being so!

Some health professionals may feel insulted and distressed when patients seek or use alternate cures or therapies, which are often dismissed as "folk medicine." Not all alternative healing systems are ineffective; some can alleviate physical symptoms, and many address psychosocial issues ignored by biomedicine. People from other cultures think that Western medicine is not always capable of curing or alleviating particular disorders or conditions, especially those caused by spirits, ancestors, or behavioral impropriety. Often, Western medical treatments and alternative or native therapies are viewed as mutually exclusive endeavors.

No matter how smart and experienced a person may be, at times of great stress, such as illness or death, early-learned ideas resurface and structure responses.

As a physician, I have learned through the years that I have to keep an open mind when it comes to finding what is best for my patients. Coming from a background where I was exposed to multiple approaches to healing, this is not difficult. I am aware that some treatment modalities, even those that appear to work, have no "scientific" backup.

Following are several alternative methods that have been applied throughout the years.

Mind-Body Interventions

In this modality, the belief is that the body and the mind are interconnected, and the mind plays a significant role in illness and healing. It also recognizes the capacity of social, economic, and familial factors to affect health. Methods that can be used to enhance mental and physical health include meditation; hypnosis; self-awareness and relaxation techniques such as deep breathing, yoga, and t'ai chi; biofeedback; guided imagery; and prayer.

Meditation: Meditation is a state of quiet contemplation. In simple meditation, a subject sits quietly and focuses the mind on a single thought. In mindful meditation, a subject sits quietly and simply witnesses whatever goes through her mind without reaction. Studies have shown that meditation causes a generalized reduction in heart rate and respiration rate. It decreases cortisol (a major stress hormone) and pulse rate, and increases alpha brain waves associated with relaxation. A recent study demonstrated that meditating 20 minutes, twice a day, can decrease blood pressure significantly. Meditation is also used to relieve stress and panic disorders. Meditators are better able to handle stressful situations and have a higher general happiness measure. Meditation has been used with success in women with breast cancer who could not take hormones to relieve their perimenopausal and menopausal symptoms.[2]

Transcendental meditation (TM), introduced by Maharishi Mahesh Yogi, has been shown to reduce high blood pressure by 50 percent. Transcendental meditation is also used to decrease anxiety, drug and alcohol abuse, and heart disease.

Hypnotherapy: Hypnotherapy is the induction of a willing subject into a state of focused concentration, described as neither wakefulness nor sleep, during which the subject is open and responsive to suggestion. Hypnotherapy has been used to relieve anxiety, promote smoking cessation, and to help with sexual problems. My friend and patient, Karen Gless, R.N., Ph.D., a marriage, family, and child counselor (MFCC), has achieved success with this modality when treating couples with sexual problems.

Deep breathing: The goal of this technique is to relax both the mind and the body. Whenever you are stressed, follow these simple steps: While comfortably seated, close your eyes, and begin taking slow, deep breaths through your mouth, filling your entire abdomen as well as your lungs, and then slowly exhaling through your nose. Meanwhile, starting at the top of your head, visualize each part of your body getting limp, proceeding down through your body until you reach your toes. Remember to remain aware of your breathing.

I often practice this technique with patients who are going through a stressful period in their lives.

Yoga: *Yoga* means "union." It is a 5,000-year-old Indian practice designed to balance mind, body, and spirit, thus promoting healing. The practice of yoga combines physical movements with breathing, which promotes flexibility and muscle strength and helps the body resist disease and injury. It has been used to relieve stress, menstrual pain, hypertension, depression, diabetes, high cholesterol, and weight loss.

Biofeedback: With biofeedback, sensors are attached to the body, which are then connected to a computer that registers electrical signals from the brain and muscles. These signals are translated into images and sound. Working with a therapist, a patient learns how to affect these signals, and eventually learns how to control stress-related maladies such as anxiety, heart disease, hypertension, and urinary stress incontinence.

Guided imagery: The power of the mind is used to evoke a positive physical response during guided use of the imagination. This results in reducing stress, slowing the heart rate, stimulating the immune system, and reducing pain.

I use this method in my practice to help patients relieve stress and decrease post-operative pain and nausea. I teach my patients, prior to their undergoing chemotherapy, to visualize the medication killing the bad cells and leaving the good cells intact.

A Patient's Story

Recently my patient Ellen was suffering from a bowel obstruction following surgery for advanced cancer of her ovaries. She was distraught when she learned that she had to have a naso-gastric tube placed through her nose into her stomach. Ellen told me that she was already overwhelmed by the thought of having cancer, and now her bowels were no longer working. I explained that her bowels were not working because they were resting after the extensive surgery and not because something was wrong with them.

When I realized that Ellen had no idea how her gastrointestinal system worked, I explained how the food enters the mouth and goes down through the esophagus, and then through the stomach to be digested. The digested food is then moved through the bowels; the important nutrients are absorbed, and what is left is evacuated through the rectum. In Ellen's case, her bowels just stopped for a while, but were still producing acid and mucous. This was why I had to put the tube in, so they could rest and heal. While explaining this to her, I was touching her, tracing the path of her intestinal tract, and gently rubbing her distended and painful belly.

I taught Ellen to do some slow and deep breathing, while tracing the same path and imagining her bowels becoming healthy and starting to move. As soon as we could hear bowel sounds, the tube could be removed. Less than 24 hours later, we were able to remove the tube, which was a record! The average bowel obstruction takes about two to three days to resolve.

Spiritual Healing, Beliefs, and Prayers

Spiritual beliefs can play a crucial part in our well-being. About 95 percent of Americans believe in God, and I strongly believe in prayer. Grandma prayed at least one hour every day. Prayers are known to bring about relaxation, hope, and comfort. A belief in what you are praying for is very important. I pray for my patients who are undergoing chemotherapy. When someone I know is going to have life-threatening surgery, I always ask for the date and exact time when the surgery will take place, and I pray during those times. Growing up in Haiti, living through many heart-wrenching situations, I believe that I survived and helped others heal because of prayer.

While I was doing obstetrics, whenever a premature baby was in neonatal intensive care, Grandma and I both prayed for the baby. The babies always did very well, regardless of how premature they were. One of them, Megan, is now a vivacious ten-year-old. She was two pounds when she was born. Whenever her mother comes for her annual exam, she always tells me that knowing that Grandma was praying for her gave her more hope.

According to the results of a recent 28-year study of 5,000 churchgoers, those who regularly attended religious services lived longer than those who did not. Those who did not attend church experienced a 36 percent higher death rate than those who did. It was theorized that this discrepancy could be explained by increased social contacts, improved health practices, more stable marriages, and perhaps, the belief in, and practice of, prayer.

According to a 1995 study at Dartmouth's Hitchcock Medical Center, one of the strongest predictors of survival after open-heart surgery was the degree to which patients said they drew strength and comfort from religion. Many studies have revealed lower rates of depression and anxiety-related illness among those who pray.

A TRUE-LIFE STORY: THE POWER OF PRAYER

One of my recent experiences having to do with the power of belief and prayer was with Gina. A 63-year-old woman, she had been my patient for many years. Her husband, a doctor, had just retired. Gina came in for her regular checkup with some vague complaints. She was happy that she could finally spend time with her husband and occasionally visit her children.

My physical exam revealed a large pelvic mass that was confirmed to be a probable ovarian carcinoma. I referred her to one of the best gynecologic oncologists in town, Dr. Steve Plaxe; we decided to operate on her as co-surgeons. When Gina realized that she was going to have surgery, she was adamant that she wanted to stay awake during the surgery. She was afraid that she would never wake up. I advised her to talk with the anesthesiologist, Dr. John Welton.

I asked her what would make the process easier for her if she did have to be put to sleep. "Maybe singing my favorite song for me while I am falling asleep," she replied. Gina's favorite song was "Mama," one of my favorite Italian songs. Since Gina had an English last name, I never knew that she was Italian! "If I have to be put to sleep, will you sing it for me?" she asked. "No, Gina," I answered. "We will sing it together." Due to the nature of her procedure, which could mean removing possible tumors anywhere in the abdomen, the anesthesiologist felt that a spinal or epidural was not prudent. Gina had to be put to sleep.

The day of the surgery, Gina was in tears when I entered the operating room. She was lying on the operating table, still begging the anesthesiologist not to put her to sleep. "Remember, we are going to sing together," I said. "Don't worry." And, as promised, we sang, *"Mama, solo per te la mia canzone vola . . ."* while she gently drifted off to sleep.

Yes, indeed, the mass in her abdomen was cancerous. I knew that she would be taking chemotherapy treatments and that her five-year survival rate was about 15 percent. I spent time with Gina and her family, teaching them about coping mechanisms; and explaining how faith, prayer, good nutrition, chemotherapy, counseling, and support groups were "a must." I told them about the "faith of the mustard seed" prayer from the *Book of Promises.* A sick person is supposed to claim his or her healing and believe that he or she has already been healed. The person might say: "Thank you, God, for healing me."

I talked with Gina's husband and son for a long time. Her children had a strong faith in God.

"Thank you, God, for healing me," Gina promised to say every time she felt overwhelmed by her disease. Her husband would say, from time to time, "Thank you, God, for healing my wife." And her children, "Thank you, God, for healing my mother."

Gina cried and cried. We talked about living one day at a time, and that the only difference between us was that she was given sort of a deadline. I could die on my way home. We all will eventually die. We just have to make the best of our life, day by day, one day at a time. Gina recovered from her surgery and continued her chemotherapy with Dr. Plaxe. Unfortunately, six months after her surgery, her mammogram showed a suspicious mass in her left breast, which turned out to be cancer. I referred her to Dr. Michael Musicant, a surgeon who is skilled with his hands and also cares greatly for his patients. The lumpectomy showed that the cancer had spread beyond the margins of the biopsy. A month later, Gina had a mastectomy. It was devastating. An assistant surgeon is not necessary for a lumpectomy, but I decided to be with Gina. I was also there for the mastectomy. We became very close.

Just before Gina's mastectomy, I met Louise Hay, who sent me a box of her inspirational books. "One set for you, and the other for some of your patients who may need them," she wrote. I gave *You Can Heal Your Life* to Gina; the book was inscribed, "From Louise, through me, to you. Remember, you have the power within you to heal yourself, one day at a time." A year later, I received this note from Gina:

Dear Dr. Carolle,

You have literally been a lifeline to me during my trials. You were by my side through three cancer operations, singing me to sleep in my native language, Italian. Each time I was going under the anesthesia, my last vision was of your caring and smiling face. When I needed encouragement through the chemotherapy, there you were telling me funny stories, urging me not to give up, and to live one day at a time. You also brought to my home a gift of the book You Can Heal Your Life, *by Louise L. Hay. All of this sustained me and saw me through my dark moments.*

Thank you, Dr. Carolle, for teaching me to have the faith of the mustard seed as in the Bible parable. It works! All my cancer tests have come back negative. You are the best doctor anyone could ever hope to have, and in the process, you have become a friend.

With much love and gratitude,
Gina

As of this writing, Gina is alive and well —and cancer free.

Alternative Systems of Medical Practice

Alternative systems can include Ayurvedic medicine, Chinese medicine (including acupuncture), and others.

Ayurvedic medicine: Ayurveda (meaning "science of life") has been practiced in India for more than 2,500 years. The belief is that the human body represents the entire universe in microcosmic form, and only by observing and understanding the world can knowledge about how the human body functions be obtained. According to Ayurveda, health is soundness and balance between body, mind, and soul, and an equilibrium between the doshas (the concept of metabolic body types). Doshas consist of the three types of biological humors: vata, pitta, and kapha, which determine an individual's constitution. There are also five elements: air, earth, ether, fire, and water. Each person contains some of the five elements. The focus of Ayurveda is prevention and healing.

Ayurvedic medicine is now known in the United States due to the efforts of Deepak Chopra, M.D., who resides in San Diego, California.[3]

Chinese Medicine

Chinese medicine uses a variety of techniques that include acupuncture, acupressure, herbal therapy, and massage to treat disorders by restoring the balance of vital energies in the body.

Acupuncture: Acupuncture is a system of medicine that has been used for over 6,000 years. Diagnosis is made by listening to the patient; observing the tongue, face, and body; taking the pulse; and palpation of indicated areas. The principle is that the cells in the body are fed by both blood and energy. The energy is called *qi* (also known as *chi*). Over the centuries, the Chinese have mapped energy channels (meridians) that flow throughout the body. It is believed that disease occurs when the flow of energy in these channels is interrupted. Needles are used to restore energy flow by stimulating specific points. This system of medicine has been used in China for all kinds of health conditions. Acupuncture has even been successful in the treatment of alcoholism.

I have personally been treated with acupuncture (after I broke my right ankle), by my friend and patient, Dr. Susan Foley, and found it to be very helpful.

Acupressure: Acupressure is also based on the concept of qi. Finger pressure, instead of needles, is employed at the same acupuncture points. This treatment can be effective, but the results from acupressure may be less dramatic than acupuncture since the points are stimulated differently.

Manual Healing Methods

The hands can be used to promote healing, too. Some examples are massage therapy and chiropractic. Touching is a powerful method of healing, which I have experienced and witnessed.

On one occasion, I had severe gastritis and could not drive myself to the pharmacy. Grandma sat at my side, praying and gently rubbing my stomach. Her healing hands were better than any antacid. I relaxed and finally went to sleep. When I woke up, I felt better.

When I have a distressed patient, I always hold her hand, or touch or rub the area where she's having pain. I hadn't realized how soothing this could be until I broke my ankle. I was lying on the emergency room's gurney when one of my colleagues, Dennis Wilcox, a surgeon, saw me. He instinctively held my hand in both of his. While he was doing so, and for a while after he left, I was in no pain.

Here are some other healing methods:

Chair massage: For the busy soul, chair massage can be performed while at work, fully clothed, and seated in a comfortable massage chair. The head, shoulders, arms, and back are massaged.

Chiropractic medicine: The basic premise of chiropractic principles is the belief that there is an innate intelligence that created our body, and it knows perfectly well how to manage and maintain it.

The system of the body most directly affected by a chiropractic adjustment is the nervous system. Chiropractic care has been well documented as an effective method for pain relief (back pain, headaches, sciatica); as well as a means of increasing spinal flexibility and integrity to maintain or activate a proper exercise regimen. The goal of chiropractic care is to assist the body in achieving its own level of optimum health.

Dr. Doreen Borseth, a chiropractor in San Diego, has been able to help some of my patients who could not take estrogen. She believes that menopause is a time of shifting hormonal regulation, and any interference within the nervous system makes return to homeostasis (the internal balancing act) that much more difficult. Chiropractic adjustment and attunement of the whole body is an effective means of restoring and maintaining balance during menopause, as well as through all of life's passages.

Massage: Massage is the systemic manipulation of soft tissue with hand strokes and occasional static pressure. Physical touch has been demonstrated to increase the rate of healing, enhance the immune system, and stimulate the body to release hormones called endorphins, which are responsible for a feeling of well-being. Massage therapy can also be used to help alleviate depression, headaches, insomnia, stress, anxiety, and tension.

Reflexology: Reflexology involves manipulation of specific areas of the feet, which correspond to particular organs or body systems that can bring the body into balance. I was introduced to reflexology by one of my patients, Sabrina Cox, who was taking reflexology classes. One day she came to my office and told me that I looked tired; she felt that I needed to relax. She returned after office hours to do a reflexology session with me. Since then, I've become hooked! Sabrina now comes to my house for the reflexology sessions. After each session, I am so relaxed that I go to sleep immediately. When I wake up the next day, I feel like a new person.

Other Therapies

Aromatherapy: Aromatherapy is the use of fragrance from essential oils extracted from plants and herbs to promote health. Aromatherapy has been used to relieve stress, depression, and insomnia, among other ailments.

Dancing: Dancing is one of the most ancient expressions of human emotion. While moving, you are relaxing, being physically creative, and releasing tension. While living in Milwaukee, I took belly dancing lessons. Then, when I was going through rough times after I moved to San Diego, I used this form of dance as an escape. And when my teacher, Athea, asked me to be one of the dancers in her teaching video, *Athea and Friends,* I only hesitated for one second. Now you know a secret: I am the tall, lanky, and beautiful belly dancer called "Akisha" in that video (which was featured on *Entertainment Tonight*)!

Lately, my love for belly dancing has been rekindled—especially now that I have regained my youthful weight and am able to fit into those gorgeous costumes of yesteryear. My husband, Albert, loves it!

Diet, nutrition, and herbal therapy: Specific foods, vitamins, and minerals can be used to prevent illness and treat disease. Herbs can have different effects on different people. Marie Kastner, a licensed acupuncturist and herbalist, graciously offered to teach me about herbs and dosages for common gynecological problems. If a patient wishes to use herbs for treatment, she should seek the help of an herbalist or a naturopathic doctor and not rely on hearsay or clerks in health food stores.

The following are some herbs and preparations that my patients have used with good results, chosen with the help of herbalists.

—*American ginseng (Panax quinquefolius):* American ginseng can help with stress, depression, fatigue, colds, respiratory problems, and damaged immune systems. It also lowers cholesterol. The recommended dosage is two capsules or 15 drops per day.

Side effects may include headaches, insomnia, anxiety, breast soreness, postmenopausal bleeding, increased blood pressure, and heart palpitations.

Caution: If you are taking hypertensive medications of any kind, do not take this herb.

— *Asian ginseng (Panax ginseng):* Panax is one of the most studied Chinese herbs. It helps increase energy; relieve stress, improve memory, and aid in concentration; and it enhances sexual desire. It also decreases cholesterol[4] and platelet stickiness, in the same way that aspirin does. The recommended dosage is two capsules, or 15 drops per day of ginseng standardized to 4 percent ginsenosides.

Side effects can include breast pain, insomnia, diarrhea, and postmenopausal bleeding, if taken in high dosages for a long period of time. Do not take it if you have high blood pressure or take an MAO inhibitor.

— *Black cohosh (Cimicifuga racemosa):* Black cohosh is available in pills, liquids, and extracts. It helps relieve hot flashes, night sweats, and vaginal dryness; and emotional symptoms such as anxiety, depression, and irritability. It is commonly used in Germany in the drug Remifemin, and it is also available in the United States.

Short-term side effects include dizziness, diarrhea, and nausea. Black cohosh produces endometrial stimulation and may cause vaginal bleeding. Because of the possible estrogenic action, it should be used with caution after six months. The recommended dosage is 10 to 15 drops, or three to four capsules per day. The long-term side effects are unknown. Avoid use if you have heart disease.

— *Chamomile (Matricaria recutita):* Chamomile helps with nervousness, sleepiness, upset stomach, restlessness, and menstrual cramps. German studies have demonstrated its anti-inflammatory and antispasmodic properties. Chamomile is sold as a prepared tea, tincture, essential oil, and fresh flower. The recommended dosage is one cup of warm tea, or four capsules at bedtime.

Side effects can include occasional allergic reactions among individuals who are sensitive to ragweed.

— ***Dong quai*** *(Angelica sinensis):* Dong quai is a Chinese plant that is available in tinctures, extracts, capsules, pills, and powders. It is made from the leaves, fruits, and roots of the plant. It relieves breast tenderness, anxiety, insomnia, and sore joints. Studies have revealed that it can help reduce hot flashes and has pain-relieving qualities. The recommended dose is two grams per day. However, one study showed that the effectiveness of dong quai in relieving menopausal symptoms was shown to be no better than a placebo.[5]

A side effect of dong quai is sun sensitivity. It is contraindicated in patients taking blood thinners, and for women with fibroids.

— ***Evening primrose oil*** *(Oenothera biennis):* To help reduce hot flashes, breast lumps, and anxiety, the recommended dosage is 500 mg, two or three times per day.

— ***Garlic*** *(Allium sativum):* Garlic is a well-recognized medicinal herb with many beneficial properties. It has a strong antifungal and antibiotic agent, and also has the ability to prevent harmful blood clotting. Garlic has been found to lower triglycerides, increase high-density lipoprotein (HDL), and lower low-density lipoprotein (LDL). It also reduces blood pressure.[6] It has been shown that most types of garlic provide general benefits, but some health-care practitioners such as Dr. Andrew Weil (author of *8 Weeks to Optimum Health*) feel that it should be consumed raw. Talk to your health-care provider before using garlic supplements if you take an anticoagulant.

— ***Ginger*** *(Zingiber officinalis):* Ginger is widely used in Japanese and Chinese cooking, and it is also used as a medicinal herb in Ayurvedic and Chinese medicine. Ginger lowers cholesterol levels and causes platelets in the blood to be less sticky. It is also well known for its anti-nausea and anti-motion sickness activity. The dried or fresh root can be used to make tea. Side effects may include heartburn.

— *Ginkgo (Ginkgo biloba):* Ginkgo biloba has been widely studied in Europe.[7] It is approved by the FDA and can be obtained as a prescription drug under the name of Bio-Ginkgo. Ginkgo acts as a vasodilator, dilating blood vessels throughout the body. It can be used to relieve short-term memory loss, improve concentration, reduce ringing in the ears, and for the treatment of Alzheimer's disease. Ginkgo comes in the form of pills and tinctures. To make sure that you're getting the right kind of ginkgo biloba, it should say "guaranteed standardized extract 3 percent" on the bottle. The recommended dose is 60 mg, two to three times per day. Side effects are minimal.

— *Hawthorn (Crataegus laevigata):* Hawthorn is thought to dilate blood vessels, thereby facilitating blood flow and lowering blood pressure. It is also recommended for the treatment of insomnia, and it is a tonic for the heart.

Side effects include a dramatic drop in blood pressure. If you take a blood pressure or heart medication, you should consult with your health-care provider before taking hawthorn.

— *Hops (Humulus lupulus):* Hops have been used in Europe for centuries for such conditions as restlessness, sleep disturbances, excitability, and nervous tension. There are no dependence or withdrawal symptoms associated with the use of hops. No side effects have been reported.

— *Kava kava (Piper methysticum):* Kava kava, a native plant of Polynesia, contains kavalactones. Kava kava is used in many Polynesian ceremonies, and also throughout the world for insomnia and anxiety. The recommended dosage is two capsules per day.

Side effects may include sleeplessness and nausea. If you are taking a barbiturate, an antidepressant, or a tranquilizer, you should not use kava kava. Do not use before driving.

— *Lady's mantle (Alchemilla vulgaris):* Lady's mantle has been used to help lessen menstrual bleeding. It supposedly works by strengthening the uterus. The recommended dosage is five to ten drops of the fresh plant tincture three times per day, one to two weeks before the menstrual cycle. Side effects are minimal.

— *Licorice root (Glycyrrhiza glabra):* Licorice root helps relieve sore joints, vaginal dryness, and hot flashes. Licorice may balance the estrogen/progesterone ratio. The recommended dosage is two capsules per meal.

Side effects can include hypertension and electrolyte imbalance.

— *Passion flower (Pasiflora incarnata):* Passion flower has been used as a digestive aid; and it also helps to relieve tension, anxiety, restlessness; and to promote sleep. Two tablespoons of the dried herb can be steeped in a cup of boiling water for 15 minutes, or use 15 to 50 drops of the extract in juice or water.

Side effects include gastric upset and sleepiness.

— *Skullcap (Scutellaria lateriflora):* Skullcap is used to calm the nervous system; and relieve stress, insomnia, and muscle tension. Skullcap can be prepared as a tea. Pour one cup of boiling water over two teaspoons of dried leaves, and steep for 10 to 15 minutes. This tea can be taken two to three times per day.

Side effects include upset stomach and occasional diarrhea.

— *St. John's wort (Hypericum perforatum):* St. John's wort helps relieve anxiety, and has been used for many years in Europe as a first-line treatment for mild depression. It may also be indicated in the treatment of moderate and severe depression.[8] It acts much like Paxil and Prozac and other selective serotonin reuptake inhibitors (SSRIs). St. John's wort should not be used with any of these drugs, or with other antidepressants. The recommended daily dosage is 300 mg, three times per day; it should not be taken for more than eight weeks at a time.

Side effects may include gastrointestinal disturbances and increased sun sensitivity in fair-skinned people. Use sunscreen while taking it, and avoid intense sun exposure.

— *Valerian (Valeriana officinalis):* Valerian root, also called English valerian or Capon's tail, is a perennial herb native to Europe that contains valeric acid. It has been used for hundreds of years as a mild sedative, and for the treatment of insomnia and anxiety. Valerian root has been approved for food use by the U.S.

Department of Agriculture (USDA). The recommended dose for insomnia is two grams *before* bedtime and another two grams *at* bedtime.

Side effects may include headaches, restlessness, fatigue, nightmares, and nausea. Valerian should not be used for more than two weeks at a time. Do not use before driving.

— ***Vitex*** *(Vitex agnus-castus):* Chasteberry tree, or vitex, is believed to create a proper balance between estrogen and progesterone. It can also be used to treat menstrual irregularities, premenstrual syndrome (PMS), and menopausal symptoms. The recommended dose is one capsule two to three times per day, or 10 to 30 drops of extract in water or juice three times per day. Side effects are minimal.

Homeopathy: The basic tenet of homeopathy is that "like cures like." This means that if you have a symptom, you choose a medicine that, in its raw form, might *cause* that symptom. Homeopathic medicines are extremely diluted substances, prepared in a nontoxic way. Homeopathy is used to treat various ailments including insomnia, headaches, and menstrual problems.

Light therapy: Research indicates that in order to stay healthy, the body needs adequate exposure to natural sunlight. Light therapy can be used to treat various ailments, including depression and insomnia, and also has been advocated for use among women with irregular bleeding to regulate their menses. However, there are no rigorous scientific studies available to back up these menopause-related claims.

Buyer Beware

There are many brands of herbal medications on the market. Because they are classified as a food, they are not regulated. Remember:

- When you're shopping, look for "standardized" ingredients. This indicates that there has been an attempt to ensure that each dose contains the same amount of active ingredients.

- Buy products that detail ingredients, dose, and manufacturer.

- Compare the Latin names to be sure which herb you're buying. Also, purchase herbs that indicate the percentage of active ingredients, and look for other chemicals that may have been used in the preparation.

- Buy the tablets, capsules, or tincture formulation that are appropriate for the herb involved.

- Over-the-counter medications can interact adversely with prescription medications you are already taking.

- Do not try to take too many supplements at one time, at first. It will be too difficult to learn which supplement may be causing a side effect and which may be helping!

- Always check with your health-care provider before taking any over-the-counter medication.

- Rely on medical research, not package claims.

How to Choose an Alternative Practitioner

As with any method, you need to work with a practitioner you can trust. Choosing an alternative practitioner requires the same steps you would use to choose a conventional practitioner. You can get a referral from a friend or doctor, or you can check the resources in the back of this book.

I suggest that you look into the practitioner's training and experience, and choose a practitioner with a diverse background—one who has the knowledge of both natural and conventional treatments, who knows the limitations of alternative approaches, and who will be willing to refer you to, or work with, a conventional practitioner. Someone with whom you share a good rapport and open communication is a good choice.

CHAPTER 3

Perimenopause

Menopause is a process that goes on for many years and is different for every woman. Perimenopause is the period preceding menopause. During this time, the ovaries begin to diminish their cyclic production of estrogen and progesterone until they stop doing so entirely. Meanwhile, menstrual periods become more irregular and infrequent, eventually ceasing altogether. Perimenopause is, in essence, a time of declining ovarian function, and may last from four to five years.[1] Menopause is defined as no menses for six months to one year.

Symptoms of Perimenopause

Perimenopause is a time of transition, and no two women experience this transition in the same way. The symptoms, and their duration and intensity, vary considerably.

About 15 to 20 percent of women barely notice any changes, but another 15 to 20 percent experience severe problems. Due to declining estrogen, women may experience any of the following symptoms: hot flashes, insomnia, anxiety, pounding heart, vaginal dryness, lack of sexual enjoyment, lack of concentration, forgetfulness, stress, and possibly irregular bleeding.

Premenstrual symptoms such as bloating, weight gain, breast tenderness, irritability, migraine headaches, anxiety, and occasional cramping may be worse during the perimenopausal years. In some women with short-ened cycles, these symptoms appear even more frequently.

Hormonal Treatment of Perimenopausal Symptoms

Hormone therapy for a symptomatic perimenopausal woman is deter-mined by her health and hormonal status, and her desire for such therapy.

Low-dose birth-control pills (the Pill) are the treatment of choice for nonsmoking women with irregular menses. The Pill can also help prevent bone loss during perimenopause. Other benefits of the Pill include a decrease in fibrocystic changes of the breast and fibroadenoma, reducing the need for breast biopsies. By regulating the menses, the Pill also reduces the need for diagnostic tests such as endometrial biopsies, dilation and curettage (D&C), and surgical procedures such as hysteroscopy (looking inside the uterine cavity), endometrial ablation (burning of the endometri-um), and hysterectomies (removal of the uterus). The Pill also offers a method of safe contraception.

A PATIENT'S STORY

My patient Jody had severe problems with PMS, irregular bleeding, and bad cramping. They all disappeared when I started her on birth-control pills at age 46. (Every six months I had to write a letter to her insurance company to let them know that the Pill was not being prescribed for birth control!) In compar-ison, HRT has only one-quarter to one-eighth the amount of estrogen and progestin as the Pill. When a woman reaches the age of 50, she should be think-ing about stopping the Pill, but when Jody reached that age, she didn't like the idea of stopping because she had been feeling so much better while on it.

Then I saw an article referencing Lynne Shuster, M.D., a Mayo Clinic internist, who said women can stay on the Pill until menopause. She felt that even staying on the Pill one or two years past menopause presented no dan-ger to a woman's health.

After reading the article, I immediately called Jody; and another patient, Ginger, age 51, who had been on the Pill to control her severe acne and was reluctant about stopping. They were both happy to hear this good news about birth-control pills.

❦ ❦ ❦

In order to stop the Pill, a follicular-stimulating hormone (FSH) level, is drawn one week after the last pill or the morning a woman begins her next pack. If her FSH is greater than 30 International Units/Liter (IU/L), it means that she is menopausal. If the Pill was also used for contraception, a barrier method of contraception should be used for the next three months after stopping the Pill to ensure infertility. The barrier method can be discontinued when a repeated FSH remains elevated.

Some women may only experience irregular bleeding without any other perimenopausal symptoms, and may be deficient only in progesterone. After an endometrial biopsy has ruled out pathology, I prescribe progesterone compounded by a pharmacist, or a synthetic progesterone, progestin. I do not recommend progesterone cream sold over-the-counter because of its low strength and product variability.

A woman does not have to wait until she is menopausal (no menses for six months to a year) to start on low-dose estrogen therapy. For a woman with regular cycles but severe hot flashes, low-dose estrogen supplements such as Estrace 0.5 mg, Estratab .3 mg and Ogen 0.625 mg, half a tablet; or a 0.025 mg or 0.325 mg patch work wonders. She can then be switched to regular estrogen replacement therapy (ERT) when she has no more periods.

A Patient's Story

My patient Shannon reluctantly came to see me at her husband's request. She was 46 years old, with a high-profile job, and had been having problems concentrating and staying focused. She was also having hot flashes and difficulty sleeping. Fatigue made her lash out at everyone in sight. Her sex life was non-existent.

Shannon's periods had been irregular, and she'd had a tubal ligation years ago. After considering a number of options, we agreed that she could benefit from Estratab .3 mg taken every day, except when she was menstruating. Three weeks later, I received a bouquet of flowers with a card. It had a picture of a dancing bear holding a daisy with the following note: "My husband, my boss, my co-workers, my friends, and myself thank you, Dr. Carolle."

Perimenopause and the Menstrual Cycle

Each month as long as you have a menstrual cycle, the female hormones FSH and LH act within an ovary to stimulate the growth of a Graafian follicle (a small sac that contains an egg), and the secretion of estrogen. This is called the follicular phase. At midpoint in the cycle, around day 14 to 15, the follicle matures and bursts, producing an egg. The follicle now shifts to the corpus luteum phase, secreting estrogen and progesterone. These hormones help the lining of the uterus, the endometrium, grow. The egg is caught by one of the Fallopian tubes, which carries it toward the uterine cavity. If the egg has not been fertilized by a sperm, it disintegrates, and the endometrium sheds in the form of menstrual blood. The beginning of the menstrual flow is considered the first day of the menstrual cycle.

Because of the hormone-production changes in the ovaries during perimenopause, approximately 80 percent of women will experience some kind of change in their menstrual cycle during these years.

Hormonal Variation and the Menstrual Cycle

Short cycles: A patient whose cycle has been 25 to 35 days may find that it changes to 21 to 24 days. Due to ovulation occurring less frequently, menstruation may occur as often as every 21 days. Cycles are shorter because there is little production of estrogen during the follicular phase.

Missed cycles: The pituitary gland increases the FSH level, attempting to stimulate dwindling follicular activity. In some cases, the follicles do respond, and estrogen and progesterone are released, resulting in a menstrual period. When the follicles do not respond, ovulation does not occur, and there is no menstrual period. Some women can miss a period or two; others may miss up to four periods, only to resume regular menstruation. The longer the time between cycles, the more likely you are to experience hot flashes, night sweats, and/or other symptoms previously discussed. As the cycles are resumed, these symptoms diminish.

Light periods: When estrogen is low, there is little stimulation of the endometrium. When bleeding occurs, it is usually very light.

Heavy periods: As follicles respond to the release of FSH, estrogen is produced, but there is no ovulation. Because ovulation does not occur, there is no production of progesterone to counteract the action of estrogen on the endometrium. Thus, the menstrual period that results may be very heavy. Copious and irregular bleeding can be very disruptive to lifestyle, and if it persists for a long time, it can cause anemia, which is the reduction of the number of red blood cells, or the reduction of the amount of hemoglobin in the blood.

Other Nonhormonal Causes for Irregular Bleeding

Underactive thyroid: In my experience, about one in ten women experiences irregular or heavy bleeding due to an underactive thyroid. Your health-care provider can rule this out by doing a simple blood test checking your TSH (thyroid stimulating hormone).

Stress: Acute or prolonged stress can affect a woman's cycle at any point in her life. Many patients have come to my office thinking they are going through early menopause. But upon further questioning, I find out the culprit is stress, especially if my patient happens to be a superwoman with a full-time job, a homemaker with small children who is earning an extra degree at night, or a similar scenario.

If my patient is under age 35, I check her TSH to make sure her thyroid is not underactive. If her TSH is normal, I recommend stress-management counseling, and ask her to reevaluate her life and come back to see me in three months. Most of the time, this is enough to regulate her menses. If the patient is over age 35, I perform an endometrial sampling in addition to testing her TSH to rule out any pathology. If there are no abnormal findings, I observe the patient for three months before initiating hormonal treatment, unless her symptoms are debilitating.

Uterine fibroids: Myomas, also known as fibroid tumors of the uterus, are almost always benign and can grow anywhere in the uterus. When their presence distorts the endometrial cavity, they can cause heavy menstrual bleeding. Fibroids are estrogen dependent; they grow with pregnancy and shrink with menopause.

Fibroids occur in more than half of all women and affect more than one-fourth of all women by age 40. Fibroids are the number one reason for hysterectomy in the U.S.[2]

Black women are three times more likely than white females to have uterine fibroids. Fortunately, there is only a .5 percent risk that fibroid tumors are cancerous.

Cervicitis: Unsuspected cases of cervicitis caused by sexually transmitted diseases such as chlamydia and gonorrhea can cause irregular bleeding. Chlamydia is transmitted by bacteria that pass from an infected person to his/her partner during sexual intercourse. Gonorrhea is an acute disease of the lining (epithelium) of the urethra, cervix, and rectum transmitted by direct genital contact. A woman infected with gonorrhea or chlamydia will notice spotting or bleeding after intercourse. A cervical culture and treatment with appropriate antibiotics will solve the problem.

Endocervical polyps: A polyp is a growth that originates from the inside portion of the cervix or endocervix and protrudes from the cervical opening. Most polyps do not cause symptoms and are discovered accidentally during routine pelvic exams. Some polyps, however, will cause abnormal vaginal bleeding following intercourse. A polyp is easily removed by grasping it with a small instrument and snipping the base with scissors.

The Pill: Currently, a good number of nonsmoking women over age 40 use birth-control pills for contraception. Taking the Pill irregularly may cause abnormal bleeding. Sometimes, after being on the Pill for many years, a patient may start to bleed irregularly. I have found that a higher-dose pill is not the answer; simply switching to a different brand generally does the trick.

Intrauterine device (IUD): An IUD is a piece of plastic partially covered with copper wire that is placed in the uterine cavity to prevent pregnancy. Some women may experience spotting between periods, or longer and heavier periods during the first few cycles following IUD insertion.

Alcohol abuse and excessive use of aspirin: Both alcohol abuse and excessive aspirin use can adversely affect the formation of platelets, which are blood cells that help the blood to clot. Blood does not clot as well with fewer platelets, leading to increased bleeding.

Pregnancy: Pregnancy can and does occur during the perimenopausal period. I learned this firsthand after I finished my residency: A 45-year-old woman who'd had a tubal ligation years ago came to my office complaining of irregular bleeding. I assumed that she was perimenopausal. Later, I got a call from the emergency room where the woman had been admitted in shock. She had a ruptured ectopic pregnancy.

❧ ❧ ❧

Other causes for irregular bleeding include cervical, tubal, and uterine cancer.

When Is Irregular Bleeding Serious Enough to Go for Help?

If you are experiencing any of the following symptoms, you should see your health-care provider:

- Bleeding that is heavier than normal, lasting an unusually long period of time, and occurring more frequently than your regular cycle.

- Bleeding between periods. Some women experience minor spotting up to two to three days before or after their period. This should not cause any concern. But if you experience bleeding similar to your period between cycles, you should be on the alert.

- Bleeding that occurs during or after intercourse.

- Bleeding that occurs after you have stopped menstruating for more than a year.

The Menstrual Calendar

During perimenopause, I recommend keeping a menstrual calendar. It is very helpful to me when a patient with irregular bleeding arrives at my office with her menstrual calendar in hand.

The Menstrual Cycle Calendar

Month_____

SUN	MON	TUE	WED	THUR	FRI	SAT

Tracking Your Menstrual Bleeding

Before using the menstrual-cycle calendar, I suggest you make several copies to use in future months, or make your marks in pencil.

On the calendar, record your level of bleeding for each day, using the following abbreviations:

- "H" = heavy bleeding (passing clots or soaking through a pad or tampon every two hours or less)

- "M" = moderate bleeding

- "L" = light bleeding

- "S" = spotting

How to Deal with Lack of Concentration and Forgetfulness

A number of my perimenopausal patients—women accustomed to being in charge of their lives—have come to my office over the years complaining of forgetfulness and lack of concentration. I did not realize how frightening this could be until one day, when I was 47, a woman approached me in a store, calling me by my first name and telling me how glad she was to see me. (People with whom I am not close usually call me Dr. Jean-Murat.) *This has to be someone I know very well,* I thought. The woman came right up to me, kissed me, and said how sorry she was that I had missed her last party. I tried in vain to remember who she was.

It took several minutes for me to realize that the woman was Marcia, a dear friend of mine! I was shocked that my brain had failed me in this way. It was an unusual and scary experience. I have had no problems remembering things that happened years ago, even when I was writing one or even two books at a time. I performed major surgery and juggled many different tasks. But the day arrived that I realized I could no longer totally rely on my memory to remind me of the things I had to do that day! It seemed to me that loss of concentration was not from lack of estrogen alone. I used birth-control pills, so I shouldn't have had a lack of estrogen. The villain had to be the aging process itself.

I now use a daily planner and review it every morning. Sticky notes lie everywhere to remind me what I need to do. At my office, I leave myself reminders on the answering machine. At home, I keep a carbon-copy message book next to my answering machine, record all messages, and leave them in full view.

Studies have shown that taking 60 mg twice a day of the Chinese herb gingko biloba is very helpful with memory problems.

Remember, memory loss can also be caused by stress, insomnia, depression, and certain medications.

Blood Tests to Check Perimenopausal Estrogen Levels

I do not routinely check a woman's estrogen level. I treat my patients according to their clinical symptoms and their desire for treatment. Estrogen levels can be erratic: They can be on their way up when a test is done, yet clinically the patient is still experiencing the estrogen deficiency that was occurring earlier. The results of these tests often just confuse my patients, so I don't usually perform them. However, if a patient has had a hysterectomy, I might order an FSH test to see if she has reached menopause (the result would be an elevated level of this hormone).

If you have not reached menopause and are reading this book, you should not wait to take steps toward a healthier life! (Please see chapter 19: "Take Charge of Your Overall Health.")

CHAPTER 4

Menopause

Natural menopause, or change of life, means the cessation of menstruation and the termination of a woman's fertile period. After menopause, the ovaries are not dead; they still produce hormones, but at a much lower level. Each year, more than two million American women enter menopause.

Once a woman enters menopause, she can be considered menopausal for the rest of her life. Most women are under the impression that there is a period commonly referred to as "postmenopausal." To be technically correct, there is no such period. Once you've achieved menopause, you will be in that stage until you die. For our purposes, we will consider *menopausal* and *postmenopausal* as interchangeable.

Natural menopause typically begins around the ages of 45 to 51; for approximately 7 percent of women, it occurs prior to age 40. In places where nutrition is poor, menopause occurs even earlier. Genes may also play a role in a woman's age at menopause. One study demonstrated that women aged 45 to 54 whose mothers had experienced early menopause had a six-fold higher probability of entering menopause early, in comparison to women whose mothers entered menopause after the age of 45.

When a woman asks me to predict when she will go through menopause, I tell her to ask her mother first. My own mother went through menopause at the age of 51. When, at the age of 46, she stopped menstruating, she thought that she had gone through menopause. It took her a while to realize that she was pregnant with her sixth and last child, my baby brother, Jacky! I have always hoped that I will go through an early menopause. Since I started to have my periods, I have been looking forward to the day when they will stop!

Premature Menopause

It has been postulated that Type 1 diabetes may be a predictor of premature menopause. Hysterectomy affects estrogen production for some patients, even when ovarian tissue is preserved.[1] Also, women who smoke become menopausal about two years earlier than women who don't.

Artificial menopause can be brought on by intensive irradiation of the pelvis or by chemotherapy for cancer in another part of the body.

Surgical menopause occurs when the ovaries are removed as part of the treatment for cancer, endometriosis, or pelvic inflammatory disease. In these cases, the symptoms of menopause are typically more intense.

Life Changes and Menopause

Life expectancy for women in the United States is now 79 years, meaning that you will live about one-third of your life after menopause. In today's world, emphasis is placed on youth, particularly for women, and menopause can be a time of anxiety and emotional devastation. After age 50—the average age of menopause—the signs of aging may become more apparent. We often hear the term "midlife crisis." I do not think this is solely related to menopause because the time when it occurs can vary. I would rather refer to it as "middle age."

During this time of life, other important life changes can also come to the forefront. If a woman has never worked outside of the home, she may feel that her life has little meaning because her children are no longer at home. Women who have built their lives around their kids may decide to go back to school or seek work now that their children are gone. On the other hand, women who have had a busy professional life may decide to slow down. Others who delayed motherhood may still have young children at home, and some women may find themselves divorced, with few skills necessary for entering the working force. Some might have older parents who need help. Self-esteem may be at a low point. Coping mechanisms for so many changes will be stretched to the limit, especially if hormonal changes are also occurring.

In my Haitian culture, women age gracefully, and aging is associated with knowledge and wisdom. I grew up looking forward to growing old and being like Grandma—loved, beautiful, wise, and respected. The opposite is true in American culture, where aging is associated with mental and physical "deterioration." I have many patients who dread the idea of growing old. No one believes me when I tell them that I look forward to going through menopause!

Different Perceptions of Menopause

How a woman views menopause depends upon her culture. For instance, there is no word for menopause in the Japanese language.[2] The Japanese diet is high in soy, so Asian women experience very few, if any, menopausal symptoms.[3]

I called my mother and asked her what menopause meant to *her*. She said, "It is a time when you do not have to worry about getting pregnant, and a time when your sex drive is the highest." She also told me that she never had any symptoms. When I asked her if she had heard about a pill that you could take for menopause, she laughed and told me that she was not surprised that, as a doctor, I could find a pill for something that was a natural process.

I also called my stepmother, Eka, because I realized that I had never heard her complain about menopause. I also called Tatante, my Aunt Audency, and a classmate, Claudy, who had gone through menopause at the age of 45. All of them said the same thing: that it was a natural life event. Eka recalled that one of her sisters had experienced some bad *"bouffees de chaleur,"* or hot flashes, but they went away after a few months, without intervention.

When I called my childhood friend Alix, an engineer who lives in Maryland, to wish him a happy 50th birthday, he told me I had to be careful how I treat him because he was now my elder! Even though he was joking, his comment reaffirmed the concept that in my culture, growing older meant attaining greater respect.

Sifting through this information, I theorize that one of the reasons why we have different perceptions about menopause is that in Haiti, our diet consists mostly of rice, beans, legumes, vegetables, fruits, plantains, roots, wild yams; and a small amount of red meat, chicken, or fish. I assume that these foods may be rich in phytoestrogens, like the diet of Asian women, making menopause a breeze for us, also, as opposed to Americans.

I remember growing up with Grandma and Tatante during their midlife years. I never heard any complaints about their being sick during their periods. Consequently, I never heard about PMS, depression, or cramps.

Perhaps their attitudes affected me. All through college, I missed only one day of school. Being sick was not an excuse to miss a day. I recall one day when I was barely able to walk to school but realized that I couldn't stay home. I learned that the brain has the capacity to focus on one thing at a time. I just had to concentrate on what was happening in class, instead of the little aches and pains that were occurring in my body.

While I was in my third year of residency, one of the male residents accused me of "being on the rag." I didn't know what he meant! He explained that during certain times of the month, I was more demanding of my junior residents. This is what happens when you grow up in a society where you are so busy doing other things that you don't have time to pinpoint changes in your behavior. Perhaps some Haitian women do suffer from PMS or mild menopausal symptoms, but they don't make a big deal out of it because there are other things that are more important to focus on. The result is a society where mind and body changes in life are considered normal. Generation after generation will view it the same way.

Conversely, in a society where people are more educated and more affluent, people seek answers and remedies for everything, instead of accepting some things as natural occurrences in their bodies. These people are at the mercy of strategic marketing, which plays on their vulnerabilities and causes them to believe that what is natural is a "disease" and must be "treated" with drugs.

In most industrialized and affluent countries, women are the prime targets of marketing and media brainwashers who want them to believe that there's something wrong with them. I don't deny that women from any culture can have severe symptoms. The problem is that these women are being told to expect these maladies, find a cure, and receive treatment "forever."

When I ask my white, middle-class, perimenopausal patients what they think about menopause, a good majority invariably say that they expect a time of hardship, which should be controlled with "some kind of intervention."

Another observation I've made is that black women do not age in the same way that white women do. Black women rarely have wrinkles or premature aging of the skin. The physical appearance of "getting old" is not so distressing in black women.

I was sharing my views with my friend and patient of many years, Sue, who is white and a few weeks younger than I am, and she remarked, "So that's what I have to look forward to? I'll look like a prune, and you'll look great!" We laughed like two young girls. "Sorry, Sue, it is your *bad* genes, and my *good* genes!"

African-American Women and Menopause

Until recently, there has been very little research done on how black women in this country view menopause. One study done in Michigan found that black women viewed it as a natural transition related to aging. Some participants said that "women have been experiencing menopause for thousands of years. It is not something that has to be 'managed.' It's a natural process." A study from Philadelphia also concluded that black women tended to view menopause as a normal stage of life.

Some of the women said that the emotional symptoms of menopause bothered them more than the physical symptoms, but preferred to use alternative treatments such as stress reduction techniques for relief.

Problems Associated with Menopause

Each woman's menopausal experience is unique and should be addressed with a personal focus. About 10 percent of women have no problems whatsoever when their menstrual periods cease, because some women still continue to produce endogenous estrogen after menopause.

Hot flashes: Reduction in estrogen production produces the "hot flashes" that women, men, and comedians invariably associate with menopause. What's not so well known is that almost one in four women never experiences them! Hot flashes—a wave of heat through the body and the sensation of burning in the neck and head—result from the change in production of female hormones by the pituitary gland. They can occur every few minutes or once or twice an hour. When they occur at night, disturbing sleep, they're called night sweats. Some women are awakened by them as many as 10 or 20 times a night, resulting in insomnia, irritability, fatigue, lack of concentration, and sometimes depression. Thyroid abnormalities may also cause hot flashes.

A friend of mine, Mary, hated the thought of moving to Alaska when her husband got transferred. When they left San Diego, she was just entering the menopausal stage. Several months later, I received a phone call from Mary. She still disliked being in Alaska but explained to me that there was an upside to being there. When she was experiencing her hot flashes, she was really quite comfortable, while her friends were complaining about the cold!

More than 75 percent of women experience hot flashes during the first few months of menopause, and 45 percent still have them after five years. I have some patients in their 60s who still experience them to some degree. Some women have no symptoms at all, or the symptoms are so mild that the women don't realize that they are entering menopause until their menstrual periods have ceased. Forty percent of menopausal women suffer from debilitating hot flashes and seek medical treatment. "The only way I feel better when I'm having hot flashes is to stick my head into the refrigerator," said Rosemary, a colleague, who also remembers her first hot flash. She was in a meeting, sipping some red wine, and began to turn as red as the wine.

Here are some effective remedies for dealing with hot flashes:

— *Ayurvedic medicine:* Ayurvedic medicine views menopause as a Pitta energy imbalance. To correct that imbalance, practitioners advise you to reduce "Type A" behaviors. Practice meditation, and avoid spicy and greasy foods, caffeine, chocolate, alcohol, and artificial ingredients.

— *Bioflavonoids:* Bioflavonoids function like weak estrogen. The average dose is 500 to 2000 mg/day in divided doses. Bioflavonoids can be found in the white pulp under the rind of citrus fruits; and in the skin of berries, cherries, grapes, and leafy vegetables.

— *Estrogen:* The majority of my patients who take estrogen after menopause report that it relieves hot flashes, irritability, vaginal atrophy, and other unpleasant symptoms within two to three weeks.

— *Exercise:* Exercise decreases FSH and LH levels.[4] The results are even better when an exercise program is initiated prior to the onset of menopause.

— *Herbs:* Women of many cultures have used herbal remedies to alleviate the discomfort of hot flashes; this is especially true for traditional Chinese medicine, where the treatment is individualized for each woman. There are no definitive studies yet that indicate which herbs work best, in what dosages, and for whom. How a woman views menopause depends upon her culture. (Please check my website at **www.drcarolle.com**, which is periodically updated for information and research results.)

Chasteberry tree, or vitex, can help with hot flashes, depression, and vaginal dryness. Dong quai can alleviate menopausal symptoms; approximately two grams per day appears safe. While taking dong quai, avoid sun exposure. Or, wear sunscreen, because psoralen's photosensitized agents can produce a skin rash.

Other herbs that can provide relief from menopausal symptoms are licorice, black cohosh, fenugreek, hops, ginseng, alfalfa seeds, and sprouts.

— *Natural progesterone:* Natural progesterone has helped many women with hot flashes. Dermal progesterone creams have been shown to reduce vasomotor symptoms in up to 80 percent of women. John Lee, M.D., the author of *What Your Doctor May Not Tell You about Menopause*, is a strong advocate of the use of natural progesterone for hot flashes.

— *Prescription drugs:* Women who are experiencing debilitating symptoms but who cannot take estrogen to relieve their hot flashes may try prescription drugs. Megestrol acetate, or Megace, is a synthetic female hormone that is usually prescribed as a treatment for breast or endometrial cancer. Megace 20 to 80 mg/day reduces hot flashes by 85 percent within 30 days. A possible increase in symptoms can occur during the first week, then taper off after two weeks. Side effects may include weight gain and irregular vaginal bleeding.

Bellergal R, a combination of ergotamine, belladonna, and phenobarbital, can help reduce hot flashes, as well as some antihypertensive medications such as Clonidine. The Clonidine patch, 2.5 g changed weekly, or Clonidine HCL 0.1 mg three times per day, produces a 50 percent decrease in hot-flash frequency. Side effects may include dizziness, dry mouth, constipation, and sleepiness. Other nonhormonal drugs that can help with hot flashes are Inderal, Aldomet, Verapamil, and Paroxetine. Paroxetine 10 to 20 mg/day appears to decrease the frequency and severity of hot flashes in breast cancer survivors by up to 75 percent. Side effects may include drowsiness and anxiety.

— *Relaxation techniques:* Relaxation techniques such as deep breathing have been shown to reduce hot flashes.[5]

— *Self-awareness techniques:* A good self-awareness technique to help you deal with hot flashes is to keep a diary in which you record your activities and what you eat and when your hot flashes occur. Your hot flashes may be more frequent or intense at certain times of the day. Learning when to expect them may bring about a feeling of control.

Also, the physical environment can also affect hot flashes. It has been demonstrated that hot flashes are less frequent in cooler climates. So, drink plenty of water! You may find that certain foods or situations provoke hot flashes. Foods to avoid if you are having hot flashes include alcohol, caffeine, and spicy foods. Nicotine increases the intensity of hot flashes, and regular exercise can help reduce them. Cotton sleepwear and bed sheets, which better absorb perspiration, can provide more comfort during sleep. Keep a small, portable fan by the bedside. You should also talk with other women who are experiencing hot flashes, and exchange practical and effective solutions for coping.

— *Soy:* Japanese women, who have a diet rich in phytoestrogen, have less heart disease, breast cancer, and menopausal symptoms.[3] (See chapter 11: "Implement a Healthy Nutrition Program.")

— *Traditional Chinese medicine:* Traditional Chinese medicine uses herbs such as dong quai and ginseng to relieve hot flashes. Another option is acupuncture. Many women have used acupuncture to decrease the frequency of their hot flashes with good results.

— *Vitamin E:* Studies done in the late 1940s documented that women who could not take estrogen and were placed on vitamin E showed marked improvement—or complete relief—from their symptoms. Unfortunately, no further studies have been done since patentable HRT was made available, due to its profitability. Vitamin E dosages range from 100 IU to 1,200 IU; the dose may be increased as tolerated. It has been advised that vitamin E be taken with selenium because they operate synergistically. Women who suffer from hypertension, diabetes, or rheumatoid heart conditions should confer with their health-care provider before taking vitamin E.

HOT FLASHES MADE EASY
(A quick summary on how to treat hot flashes)

- Take vitamin E
- Exercise regularly
- Look into Ayurvedic medicine
- Use herbs; eat soy products
- Avoid stimulants

- Practice relaxation and self-awareness techniques
- Take estrogen and/or progesterone
- Get acupuncture
- Take bioflavonoids or prescription drugs

Emotional Changes and Menopause

A patient, Marla, who'd had no periods for three months, came to see me in tears. "Doc, you have to do something to help me. Lately, I have been called the 'speed witch.' I can turn from normal to a witch in less than five seconds, and I cry about everything." All of her symptoms disappeared after she began taking estrogen.

Headaches, irritability, dizziness, and heart palpitations have not been found to be directly related to lowered levels of estrogen. However, hot flashes can cause sleep deprivation, which can make you feel tired, moody, and irritable. Some women have reported fuzzy thinking and headaches. If these symptoms can be attributed to estrogen deficiency, estrogen replacement may reverse or prevent them.

Among women with increased irritability, nervousness, depression, anxiety, and headaches, a diet rich in phytoestrogens and an exercise regimen is recommended. You should also avoid caffeine and alcohol, and practice mental relaxation techniques. Acupuncture, and herbs such as ginseng, kava kava, and hops, can work wonders. Otherwise, short-term estrogen therapy plus testosterone can be tried. If each of these therapies fails, short-term tranquilizer therapy may alleviate the problem.

Other herbs that may help with anxiety include skullcap, chasteberry, passion flower, valerian root, chamomile, catnip, and peppermint tea.

Depression and Menopause

There is little evidence that estrogen deprivation causes major psychotic disorders. Women with a prior history of depression are, however, more likely to have a recurrence during menopause. (See chapter 10: "Stress and Depression.")

Sleep and Mood Disturbances

A lack of estrogen can disturb a woman's normal sleep cycle, resulting in insomnia, fatigue, and depression. These symptoms are not always attributed to the lack of estrogen. Insomnia can also be due to stress and medications.

To prevent insomnia, avoid stimulants such as caffeine and alcohol, especially late in the day. Exercise no later than three hours before bedtime. Keep the bedroom temperature comfortable, and only use this room for sleeping—not for watching television or reading and relaxing. Go to bed at the same time each night, and don't watch the clock. If you can't sleep, leave the bedroom, then return and try again when you feel tired.

Herbal therapies to reduce insomnia include valerian root, chamomile, passion flower, and hops. Chamomile, lemon balm, and lemon verbena together make a delicious tea to promote sleep. Calcium and magnesium, one tablet each, taken 45 minutes before bedtime, can have a tranquilizing effect.

Melatonin is used by millions of people as a sleep aid. How much is enough is mere speculation. Either 1 mg or 3 mg doses is recommended, and it is sold at health-food stores. A study done by the Massachusetts

Institute of Technology (MIT) in Cambridge, Massachusetts, concluded that .3 mg alone can induce sleep. However, melatonin may promote nightmares, cause nausea, and exacerbate depression.

According to J. Brooks Hoffman, M.D., a retired physician from Greenwich, Colorado, if you force yourself to yawn and keep yawning, by the sixth yawn or so, you'll likely start to feel drowsy.

I rarely prescribe prescription drugs for sleep. If your doctor agrees to do so, these medications should not be taken for more than three weeks at a time, as they can become habit-forming.

SLEEP DISTURBANCES MADE EASY

(A quick summary on how to treat sleep disturbances)

- Take estrogen and/or progesterone
- Exercise regularly
- Do body work
- Practice mind/body medicine
- Take calcium and magnesium

- Avoid stimulants
- Try melatonin
- Use aromatherapy
- Engage in stress-reduction techniques
- Take herbs and/or prescription drugs

Vaginal Atrophy

A lack of estrogen causes the uterus, cervix, and cervical and vaginal glands to atrophy, or wither, thus producing less lubricating mucus. The vagina may also lose its elasticity. A Swedish research study revealed that 39 percent of postmenopausal women reported some vaginal discomfort, 18 percent of which was moderate to severe. However, many women do not experience vaginal dryness following menopause.

Atrophic vaginal tissues are also more prone to vaginal ailments, such as yeast and bacterial infections. Estrogen is one of the quickest and most effective means to relieve vaginal atrophy. Women who are on estrogen replacement therapy (ERT), either oral or transdermal, typically do not experience vaginal dryness.

For women with symptomatic vaginal dryness who do not want to use estrogen systemically, or who are using ERT and still have vaginal dryness, I recommend trying Premarin, Estrace, or estriol vaginal cream. The amount of estrogen absorbed through the skin is negligible; the amount may be higher during the first few weeks due to the thinness of the vaginal tissue. After the vaginal tissue thickens, the amount of estrogen absorbed is minimal. I recommend applying one-third of an applicator at bedtime for one week, followed by one-third of an applicator every other night, then one-third of an applicator once or twice a week. Estring, a ring of estradiol, which is not absorbed systemically and lasts about 90 days, is also available.

Estriol vaginal cream, 0.5 mg/gram, can also be mixed for you by a compounding pharmacist. The recommended dosage is one gram ($^1/_4$ tsp) at bedtime for one week, then three times weekly thereafter. Some women do very well using only lubricants such as K-Y Jelly, Lubrin, Moist Again, Replens, vitamin E oil, and Astroglide, especially before intercourse, to keep the vagina healthy and less prone to infection; and make vaginal penetration more comfortable.

Dr. John Lee recommends transdermal natural progesterone, without estrogen, for the treatment of vaginal dryness.[6] Sometimes I recommend vaginal estrogen cream for patients who have had breast cancer and are afraid of any kind of estrogen, but whose vaginal atrophy makes their sex life miserable. One such patient, Lorna, a 55-year-old female, stopped her estrogen replacement therapy when she was diagnosed with breast cancer. Lorna had been trying many different alternative regimens and lubricants; none worked. Her younger boyfriend lived in Chicago, and they would see each other about once a month. After each encounter, her infection would recur. When I saw her, her vagina was very atrophic and infected. She did not want to use estrogen cream. After her third visit in less than three months, I again mentioned the use of transvaginal estriol cream. Lorna finally agreed. Since then, her problem has been resolved.

Alternative Treatments for Vaginal Dryness

Alternative treatments for vaginal dryness include herbs such as motherwort tincture, dong quai, black cohosh, and licorice, which have been found to be helpful. Vitamin E, applied inside the vagina and around the labia in oil or suppository form, can alleviate vaginal dryness as well.

To avoid vaginal dryness, it's best to avoid substances that produce a decrease in vaginal moisture, such as alcohol, caffeine, diuretics, and anti-histamines. One young patient came to my office complaining of severe vaginal dryness; six months prior to her symptom onset, she had been using antihistamines consistently due to allergies.

VAGINAL DRYNESS MADE EASY
(A quick summary on how to treat vaginal dryness)

- Take vitamin E and/or herbs
- Use lubricants
- Take estrogen and/or progesterone
- Engage in continued sexual activity
- Avoid alcohol, caffeine, and antihistamines

Menopause and Memory Problems

During menopause, some women do experience memory lapses; how-ever, this problem may be associated with allergies, thyroid disorders, and poor mental habits. Memory loss, associated with an acute decrease in estrogen, appears to be temporary.

Estrogen replacement therapy can help with memory problems. Some researchers from Canada demonstrated that women who were taking estro-gen performed better on several memory tests.

One recent study documented that extract of ginkgo biloba, used for dementia, helped to improve cognitive performance and social functioning for six months to a year. The dose used was 40 mg, three times per day. Many women have realized great improvement using ginkgo biloba, 60 mg, twice a day.

Other herbs that may be helpful include ginseng, gotu kola (*brahmi* in India), hawthorn—also known as English hawthorn—and may bush, all of which work by dilating blood vessels and improving circulation.

MEMORY LOSS MADE EASY
(A quick summary on how to treat memory loss)

- Stay mentally active
- Take estrogen and/or progesterone
- Use herbs

Menopause and Skin Problems

Katherine, a 52-year-old patient, came to my office because she was experiencing many menopause-related symptoms. Apparently, while seated in the waiting room, she began a conversation with another patient regarding her symptoms. She could not help but notice the facial hair on the woman she was speaking to. That patient had been menopausal for three years and was on hormonal replacement therapy.

Her first words to me were: "Dr. Jean-Murat, am I going to grow hair on my face like the woman in the waiting room?" I explained to her that the previous patient, Evelyn, had excessive facial hair that was completely unrelated to menopause.

Katherine was relieved to learn that women do not grow actual beards when menopausal! Throughout a woman's adult life, the ovaries do produce some testosterone, the male hormone. During menopause, the production of testosterone is reduced by two-thirds, but since the production of estrogen becomes minimal, the body produces relatively more testosterone. This explains why some women display signs of masculinization, such as a deeper voice or increased hairiness. There can also be a thinning of hair. As you age, your skin will change somewhat, but again, it hasn't been proven that menopause is the direct cause. The skin grows thinner and loses its elasticity, resulting in wrinkling. Some of this is due to a reduction in the skin's collagen content. Black women have fewer wrinkles because of the abundance of melanin and the thickness of their skin. (I call it a *blessing*.)

Wrinkles are not an inevitable part of aging! People who are exposed to the sun or who smoke over prolonged periods are much more prone to premature aging of the skin. Fair-skinned people are more vulnerable to wrinkles.

Aging of the skin depends upon race and genes. In my family, the older we get, the younger we look. I tell my envious white patients and friends that we are like wine—the older the better. I had never paid much attention to wrinkles until one day, when Grandma and I were shopping, she asked me to buy her a jar of Noxzema. I asked her why she needed it, and she told me she'd been watching television and had seen a Noxzema commercial featuring a beautiful young woman. I was a little perplexed, since Grandma spoke no English and generally never wore makeup. She was convinced that the Noxzema would help her get rid of her wrinkles. I took a good look at Grandma's 80-year-old face; the wrinkle she was concerned about was a natural laugh line. "Are you getting vain in your old age?" I asked her. "You do not need any cream; you were born with these lines."

Recently, I was invited to be a guest speaker for a group of black professional women. The discussion centered around the difficulties involved in their daily lives. I wanted them to understand that, in spite of the trials and tribulations they encountered daily, they had a precious gift. I told them a little story:

> One day God came to Earth to visit a group of black women. "I know what you are going through," God said. "In the scheme of things, others may place you at the bottom of the totem pole. To make up for this, I am going to bestow a great gift upon you. It is the gift of ever-lasting beauty. While others grow old like prunes, your skin will always be youthful. You will be the envy of all the races. You will not have to spend your hard-earned money on wrinkle creams or plastic surgery."

The sisters were smiling and laughing by the time I reached the end of that story!

The Urinary Tract and Menopause

Urinary problems can be experienced more frequently during menopause. Estrogen maintains the functional tone of the mucosa (lining) of the bladder and the urethra. Estrogen deficiency causes changes in the structure of both organs; and may result in painful urination, urinary urgency and frequency, urinary stress incontinence,[7] and a greater incidence of urinary tract infections.

Urinary incontinence, or the involuntary loss of bladder control or inability to predict when and where urination will occur, is a common disorder that affects as many as half of all women during their postmenopausal years.

Treatment of urinary stress incontinence: Dr. Arnold Kegel invented the pelvic-floor exercises, also known as the Kegel exercises, during the 1950s. This exercise involves contracting the muscles that regulate and stop urine flow. To locate these muscles, try to stop your urine flow while using the toilet.

Doing Kegel's exercises regularly can result in a decrease in incontinence and an increase in muscle strength. To do the Kegel exercises, tighten your muscles, without lifting your buttocks, and hold for 10 to 15 seconds, then release. In the beginning, you may have to do them for a shorter period of time, then increase when your muscles become stronger. Rest for at least ten seconds between each contraction, and repeat 10 to 15 times, three to five times a day, or as often as you can while driving or watching television. It's the repetition that is most important! Make sure that each contraction is as hard as you can manage. It is a good habit to contract these muscles prior to coughing, sneezing, or nose-blowing. During the Kegel exercises, be aware of using your stomach, buttocks, or leg muscles. While squeezing your muscles, place your hand on your abdomen. If you feel it move, you are using these muscles, too. The object is to isolate and use only your pelvic muscles. Pelvic-floor exercises have been found to improve the intensity of sexual response.

Some other ways to treat urinary stress incontinence are:

— **Biofeedback:** Biofeedback has been used with some success in the treatment of urinary stress incontinence.

— **Pessaries:** While you are waiting for more conservative treatments to work, you may consider using a pessary that can be fitted by your health-care provider.

Pessaries are devices made of rubber or plastic that are inserted into the vagina of women with vaginal or uterine prolapse. They include the:

- incontinence ring;
- Cube Athletic Support pessary for women who experience incontinence during rigorous exercising; and the

- Hodge Incontinence Pessary for women with small vaginal openings.

— *Incontinence shields:* The CapSure Continence Shield, when placed over the urethral opening, creates a mild vacuum that helps to control urinary loss.

The Reliance Urinary Control Insert, a soft foam triangle with gel on the back, is directly applied to the urethra to stop incontinence. The device is removed and discarded upon urination.

Femassist is a suction cup device, lasting one to two weeks, which fits over the urethra.

The pessaries and shields can be an alternative to pads and diapers while awaiting permanent treatment.

— *Surgery:* Surgery for urinary stress incontinence can be very successful. One surgical procedure includes the injection of collagen or Teflon into the urethra.

Conclusion

As you can see, the choice to be treated or not for menopausal symptoms is yours. I have always recommended that my patients be treated if they are experiencing severe symptoms. The use of estrogen therapy, when carefully chosen, usually produces relief over a short period of time. It hurts me to see patients who have severe symptoms but refuse treatment due to unfounded fears or misinformation. Unless a patient has an absolute contraindication for estrogen, or if the patient is experiencing side effects, she should use estrogen until her symptoms have resolved, and if she chooses to, slowly taper off. (See chapter 5: "Hormonal Replacement Therapy.")

The time to exercise caution with HRT is when it is used to prevent cardiovascular disease, osteoporosis, or to reduce the risk of developing breast cancer. These subjects will be covered in more depth in subsequent chapters so that you can learn about the risks, and make the right decisions for *you!*

❧ ❧

CHAPTER 5

Hormonal Replacement Therapy (HRT)

Menopause is too often referred to as a "disease" that needs to be medically treated. This trend was begun by Dr. Robert A. Wilson, a New York gynecologist who launched a 1960s crusade to "rescue" women by preaching estrogen therapy from "puberty to grave."[1] His influence was not merely confined to the United States; effects could be seen throughout Europe. Estrogen replacement therapy (ERT) was fashionable during the 1960s and into the 1970s, when complications such as endometrial cancer finally became apparent. The use of ERT declined, but it regained momentum when some studies demonstrated that by adding a progestin, a synthetic form of progesterone, the therapy could actually decrease the risk of endometrial cancer.

When estrogen is taken alone, it is called ERT. When a combination of estrogen plus a form of progesterone is used, it is called hormonal replacement therapy, or HRT. Estrogen promotes the growth of the endometrium, the uterine lining, which can increase the risk of uterine cancer.[2] A woman with an intact uterus should also be given progestin or progesterone to counteract the effects of estrogen on the endometrium.

HRT

Who is using HRT? Although estrogen therapy is widely prescribed, overall compliance is less than 30 percent. Fewer than 40 percent of American women have ever received a prescription for HRT. About one-third of women never get the prescription filled. Twenty percent of women who begin estrogen therapy discontinue it after only nine months, and 10 percent of women take their estrogen intermittently. This is mostly due to fear of the resulting side effects. Only 8 to 12 percent of postmenopausal women remain on HRT for two or more years.[3] Hormone use is most prevalent among women who are educated, Caucasian, have partners, make middle- to upper-class incomes, and who live in the midwestern United States.

— *African-American women and HRT:* The Center for Disease Control and Prevention discovered that black women were 60 percent less likely than white women to have ever taken HRT. Black women who did use it did so for a shorter period of time. This difference was found at all educational levels.

In a study in Philadelphia, it was demonstrated that black women preferred nonprescription remedies to relieve menopausal symptoms. These women also tended to view medical interventions as intrusive. In this same study, white women had a tendency to view menopause as a medical problem and were more likely to seek treatment from a healthcare provider.

Benefits of HRT

Estrogen can be helpful in decreasing short-term menopausal problems, such as hot flashes, night sweats, vaginal dryness, mood swings and other emotional changes, irritability, and depression. When a woman comes into my office complaining of severe hot flashes and other vasomotor symptoms, I typically recommend estrogen, which will resolve these symptoms within two to three weeks. Women with vaginal atrophy that impedes sexual intercourse often see a noticeable improvement within three to four weeks. For women who have had premature menopause, perhaps due to the surgical removal of their ovaries, estrogen can help relieve the acute symptoms of estrogen loss.

HRT and skin: HRT has been found to improve the elasticity of the skin. HRT can also improve its appearance by increasing its thickness and collagen content.

HRT and osteoporosis: Estrogen may be of help to women who have a strong family history of osteoporosis, or who already have osteoporosis. When there is a lack of estrogen due to a prolonged absence of menses, or following menopause, an acceleration of bone loss has been documented. Estrogen helps bones absorb calcium from the blood and slows the loss of calcium from the bone. Research has revealed that estrogen replacement can halt or slow the loss of bone mass among postmenopausal females.[4] Some studies have revealed increased bone density measurements when estrogen is taken, even if begun several years after the onset of menopause.

Data from some epidemiologic studies suggests that estrogen can also prevent fractures.

HRT and heart disease: Many observational studies have indicated that women who take estrogen for several years after the onset of menopause have a 35 to 50 percent reduced risk of cardiovascular disease. A more definitive conclusion will not be available until the year 2005 when the results of the Women's Health Initiative study will be available. The consensus seems to be that estrogen's protective effects against heart disease may be beneficial for menopausal women who have no contraindications for its use.

HRT and secondary prevention of heart attack: Many observational studies conducted with young, healthy women found a reduced risk of heart disease in women who take postmenopausal estrogen than those who did not. Observational studies also showed that there was a significant decrease in women with heart disease who took estrogen. Should HRT then be given to older women with a cardiac condition to prevent a secondary heart attack? These results have not been confirmed in clinical trials.

According to the Heart and Estrogen Replacement Therapy Study (HERS) published in August 1998, in the *Journal of the American Medical Association (JAMA),*[5] HRT, a daily dose of Premarin 0.625 mg, and Provera 2.5 mg given to older women, increased the risk of a secondary heart attack by 50 percent after the first year. There was also an increased risk of thromboembolic events (blood clots) and gallbladder disease. But by the fourth year of treatment, that risk decreased by 40 percent.

The researchers are not sure what caused these conflicting results. Now the recommendation is that HRT should not be prescribed for the purpose of preventing heart attacks in women already suffering from heart disease. However, it could be appropriate for women already receiving HRT to continue.

HRT and strokes: There are no definitive answers regarding ERT and strokes. Study results have been mixed; some show a small decrease in the rate of strokes, while some show no effect. (Please check my website at **www.drcarolle.com,** periodically updated for information and research results.)

Other Benefits of HRT

Estrogen has been found to have multiple actions in the brain that may have an important effect on Alzheimer's disease. Other benefits include a 70 percent reduction in current users, and a 40 percent reduction in former users, with respect to the risk of macular degeneration, the leading cause of blindness in the U.S. HRT may decrease osteoarthritis and tooth loss, but more research is needed.

A large study of women using HRT documented a significant decrease in colon cancer; however, the incidence of rectal cancer remained the same.

Risks of HRT

When estrogen is taken orally, its action on the liver may possibly increase the risk of gallstones and thromboembolic disease (blood clots). There may be an increase in the size of uterine fibroids among women who had fibroids before menopause. Rarely, endometriosis, a condition where tissues normally present in the lining of the endometrial cavity are found in the pelvic cavity, may be reactivated with estrogen therapy, causing irritation, pain, and scarring.

HRT makes a mammogram harder to read. There is a 25 to 30 percent increase in breast density among women taking HRT.

The Nurses' Health Study discovered that past or current estrogen users experienced a 50 percent greater risk of being afflicted with asthma than women who never took HRT.

Other HRT Risks

HRT and breast cancer: There is an increased risk of developing breast cancer for estrogen users, especially among those taking estrogen for longer than five years. (See chapter 8: "Breast Cancer: A Woman's Worst Fear.")

HRT and ovarian cancer: HRT may be associated with an increased risk of ovarian cancer.[4]

HRT and endometrial cancer: There is no clinical evidence that HRT use adversely affects women who have had endometrial cancer. Women who have had positive nodes should exercise extreme caution with HRT; there are many studies pending that will hopefully shed more light on this issue.

Vaginal bleeding and HRT: Vaginal bleeding is one of the most disturbing side effects of HRT, and occurs in 80 to 90 percent of women who use cyclic HRT. The bleeding is predictable, and of short duration, when compared to a woman's menstrual cycle.

Continual therapy was started when many women began to complain about having a monthly cycle while on cyclic HRT. These women typically experience irregular bleeding and spotting early in the treatment, which diminishes for most women within the first year. About 60 to 80 percent of women bleed while on combination therapy, and will continue to bleed for six months to a year, and 60 to 70 percent experience breakthrough bleeding or spotting.

The recommended dosage of medroxyprogesterone acetate, continuous regimen, is 2.5 mg per day. I have found that for women who have just gone through menopause, taking 5 mg per day is more effective in reducing breakthrough bleeding. When there is no more bleeding for over a year, I switch them to 2.5 mg. I have been using micronized progesterone either orally or transdermally for only a few years; it appears that these women are less likely to have vaginal bleeding.

When a woman switches from a cyclic regimen to a continuous regimen, she may experience irregular bleeding. Some women get tired of the irregular bleeding and switch back to the cyclic regimen, where they can predict the time of bleeding.

Many patients who switch to the micronized progesterone have less bleeding and other side effects.

Side Effects of HRT

Some women may experience weight gain due to fluid retention, and others may feel lower abdominal bloating. Some women with a history of migraine headaches may experience recurrences. By substituting oral estrogen with transdermal estrogen patches, many of these women will realize some relief from these side effects. Rarely, some women experience slight nausea, and others may experience mood swings.

Estrogen replacement may cause some breast pain; low doses of estrogen and androgens have been successful in reducing this breast pain. Other side effects that women may experience are leg cramps, nipple sensitivity, acne, and skin pigmentation changes.

HRT and weight gain: Women who decide to start HRT are usually concerned with potential weight gain. According to a three-year study by the National Heart, Lung, and Blood Institute, women who were taking a placebo actually gained slightly more weight than the women who were taking HRT.

Types of Estrogen for Replacement Therapy

Estrogens can be divided into three types: estrone (E1), estradiol (E2), and estriol (E3). Estradiol is the most potent and is converted into estrone in the gastrointestinal tract. Estrone has a mid-range potency. Estriol is the least potent of all estrogens.

Wild yams and other plants contain numerous hormone precursors, and when chemically processed, are transformed into synthetic hormones (estrone, estradiol, estriol, progesterone, and testosterone) that are molecularly identical to human estrogen. Estrogen can also be extracted from pregnant mares' urine, as in the case of Premarin (conjugated equine estrogen, or CEE). Many women have objected to taking Premarin because of its source; however, Premarin is still the most common oral estrogen prescribed in the United States. Most estrogen therapy studies have been done with Premarin.

Oral estrogen comes in the form of micronized estradiol (Estrace), esterified estrogen (Estratab), and piperazine estrogen sulfate (Ogen). Transdermal estrogen patches come in the form of estradiol (Climara, Vivelle, Alora), or 17 beta-estradiol (Estraderm). An estrogen gel in an alcohol base, and implants, are made of estradiol and are not available in the U.S.

Estriol: Some women who choose to use HRT are requesting estriol because they believe it to be safer than other types of estrogens. Women who live in countries with a low incidence of breast cancer typically have a higher estriol urinary excretion when compared to women who live in the U.S. and Britain, which have a high incidence of breast cancer. Asian women have higher levels of estriol.

The true effectiveness of estriol is unclear. It is appropriate for controlling menopausal symptoms, but there are no definitive studies that recommend an exact dose to prevent heart disease and osteoporosis. Current speculations are that high doses (12 mg) may be required to prevent osteoporosis. Estriol may have no effect on cholesterol.

Please refer to Part III for the table describing types and sources of estrogen (Table 20-a).

Choosing the HRT Form That's Right for You

Not all estrogens are the same. The way in which estrogen is delivered does make a difference. If you have decided to use estrogen for short-term relief of symptoms, regardless of the source, any form of estrogen will work. If your decision is long-term prevention, you should be aware of what each form has to offer and the possible side effects, which may involve experimentation. You need to choose the form that you are most comfortable with—the one that is acceptable to you and your health-care provider.

Oral estrogens: Oral estrogen is taken every day, or cyclically starting the first day of the calendar month and stopping on the 25th. I have several patients who have been taking estrogen for years, and are very happy with it. For women who still have a uterus, a progestin, most often Provera, 5 to

10 mg; or a micronized progesterone, 200 mg, is added on the 12th or the 13th day of the month and taken until the 25th day of the month. A few patients take an estrogen pill every day and add progestin or progesterone during the first 12 to 13 days of the calendar month.

Please refer to Part III for the table describing oral estrogen (Table 20-b).

Transdermal estrogens: Estrogen can also be administered through the skin using a patch (transdermal). The patch should be placed on a clean area of the buttocks or lower abdomen, and is replaced once or twice a week according to directions.

Transdermal estrogens are absorbed into the bloodstream, bypassing the liver. This form is better for women with gallbladder disease, increased triglycerides, migraines, and hypertension, or for those who suffer gastrointestinal symptoms or nausea when taking estrogen orally.

Side effects of this form include itching and skin irritation in 5 to 10 percent of users. Using a different body site each time, and waving the patch before application to make some of the alcohol evaporate, can decrease this problem.

Transdermal estrogen patches may also be less beneficial than tablets because they do not produce the favorable effect on blood cholesterol levels. More studies are necessary to discover whether transdermal estrogen offers any protective effects against heart disease in the long run.

Please refer to Part III for the table describing transdermal estrogen patches (Table 20-c).

Estrogen preparations from a compounding pharmacy: The following estrogen cream preparations can be obtained at a compounding pharmacy. (See the Resources section at the end of this book.)

- Tri-est 2.5 mg/gm (roughly the equivalent of Premarin 0.625 mg)($1/4$ tsp) transdermal cream 10% estrone (0.25 mg) 10% estradiol (0.25 mg 80% (estriol 2 mg) 60 gm –$1/4$ tsp at bedtime.

- Tri-Est 5 mg/gm (roughly the equivalent of Premarin 1.25 mg) transdermal cream 10% estrone (0.50 mg) 10% estradiol (0.50 mg 80% (estriol 4 mg) 60 gm –$1/4$ tsp at bedtime.

Vaginal estrogen creams: If the primary goal is to treat vaginal dryness, which causes pain during intercourse, estrogen cream can be a good choice. The estrogen within the cream is readily absorbed during the first few weeks, when the vaginal mucosa is atrophic. Afterward, the level of estrogen absorption is diminished. A study measured the amount of estrogen found in the blood and revealed a minimal amount, making it safe for women who are afraid to take estrogen or who may have a history of severe vaginal atrophy that does not respond to other treatments.

Please refer to Part III for the table describing estrogen vaginal creams (Table 20-d).

Vaginal ring: Estring is a soft vaginal ring that releases a low, continuous dose of estradiol over a period of 90 days. Since the amount of estrogen absorbed through the skin is minimal, the ring does not relieve other symptoms such as hot flashes, mood swings, or lack of concentration. Side effects are minimal.

Estrogen injections: Estrogen injections are used in rare cases when a woman cannot tolerate any other form of estrogen. I also use an estrogen injection immediately for a young patient whose ovaries have been removed.

I have only one patient on injectable estrogen, Janice, a 48-year-old woman. When Janice first came to see me, I suggested she try the newest oral estrogen, then the patch. After a few months, Janice demanded that I put her back on her injectable drugs. She told me that she had tried the other forms to be nice, but that they had caused one of the most miserable times of her life. I readily agreed to start her back on the injections.

Please refer to Part III for the table describing estrogen injections (Table 20-e).

Contraindications of HRT

Estrogen is not for everyone. The following is a list of absolute and relative contraindications of estrogen replacement. An absolute contraindication means you should not take estrogen if you have any of the following conditions. A relative contraindication means that you may or may not be able to take estrogen.

Absolute contraindications to estrogen therapy:

- Undiagnosed vaginal bleeding
- Acute deep venous thrombosis or evolving thromboembolism
- Current breast cancer
- Current endometrial cancer
- Acute liver disease

Relative contraindications to estrogen therapy:

- Chronic liver disease
- Endometriosis
- Fibrocystic breast disease
- Family history of high cholesterol
- Gallbladder disease
- History of breast cancer
- History of endometrial cancer
- History of deep vein thrombosis
- History of stroke or recent heart attack
- Hypertension aggravated by estrogen
- Large uterine fibroids
- Migraines aggravated by estrogen
- Pancreatic disease

Side Effects of Progestins

Some women on HRT experience symptoms related to progestins. These symptoms can include fluid retention, bloating, mood swings, depression, breast tenderness, increased appetite, and headaches. Most of these symptoms are eliminated with natural progesterone.

Risks of progestin/progesterone therapy: Another study, published in the *New England Journal of Medicine* in 1994, revealed that the addition of a progestin seemed to have a negative effect on blood cholesterol levels.

There was some concern that adding progestin to estrogen therapy for the prevention of endometrial cancer could negate the cardioprotective effects of estrogen. Evidence from the PEPI Trial in 1995,[6] and the Nurse's Health Study, demonstrated that this did not appear to be so. However, another study concluded that HRT had a persistent protective effect on the heart, but both natural and synthetic progesterones blunt the beneficial effects of estrogen on the lipoprotein profile: micronized progesterone was not superior to medroxyprogesterone acetate.[8] So the jury is still out.

Buyer Beware

Many women want to use "natural progesterone" and are using over-the-counter progesterone creams along with their ERT. You should be aware of the following:

- Creams with diosgenin from wild yam extract (which is not the same as natural progesterone cream), black cohosh, fenugreek, or other herbs that contain progesterone precursors are being touted as natural progesterone cream. The human body does not have the enzyme to convert the vegetable substances into progesterone.

- The minimal amount of progesterone to be contained in a cream to be effective is 400 mg of progesterone per ounce. Creams that have been found to contain this amount are: Bio Balance, PROGEST-1 Complex, OstaDerm, Serenity, Pro-Balance, Progonol, Pro-Gest, Pro-Oste-All, PhytoGest, Edenn Cream, Equilibrium, Estro-All, Femarone-17, Happy PMS, NatraGest, Pro-Alo, Pro-G, Angel Care, and Renewed Balance.

- It is not recommended to use over-the-counter progesterone cream in place of oral progesterone, or progestin in HRT, since the effect of those creams has not been studied.

Androgen Therapy

There is a belief that a woman loses her sex drive after menopause. This is true in some cases, but not all! Some women find that after menopause, their sexuality remains the same or even increases. Testosterone also appears to have a beneficial effect only for women whose testosterone level is low to begin with. This is the case among young women who have had both ovaries removed. Testosterone does improve sexual desire and a sense of well-being.

Adding testosterone may enhance sexual activity and satisfaction in postmenopausal women, more than adding estrogen alone. (See chapter 17: "Sexuality and the Mature Woman.")

Some data suggests some potential benefits from androgen therapy in postmenopausal women who are experiencing a decreased libido, reduced cognitive function, and the loss of their sense of well-being. In some instances, I recommend testosterone to women whose vasomotor symptoms are not responding to low-dose estrogen therapy, instead of increasing estrogen, generally with good results.

Testosterone and estrogen together may result in greater improvement in bone density than what is achieved with estrogen alone.

Side effects of androgen therapy: Possible side effects include agitation and/or depression with higher doses. It can also produce masculinization side effects, such as the growth of facial hair, acne, an enlarged clitoris, and muscle weight gain.

Risks of androgen therapy: Testosterone may also decrease HDL. These effects disappear when treatment is stopped. The Nurses' Health Study suggests that there may be an increased risk of breast cancer among women taking testosterone supplementation. The safety of taking testosterone for long periods of time has not been established.

Types of testosterone supplements: Testosterone comes in tablets of 10 mg, and sublingual lozenges of 5 mg to be broken in half and used three days a week.

Combined estrogen and testosterone pills: Testosterone is available in two combination pills with estrogen. Estratest HS is the equivalent of Premarin 0.625 mg, and Estratest is the equivalent of Premarin 1.25 mg.

Transdermal testosterone: Testosterone is also available as a transdermal cream or gel, in a variety of strengths. It can be applied to large areas of the body such as the thighs, abdomen, and arms, and is recommended for women who may need to avoid possible liver complications.

The cream or gel can be made by a compounding pharmacist. I usually start with the lowest dose and increase as necessary in order to avoid possible side effects. The recommended dose of natural testosterone gel is 10–20 mg/cc, applied daily to the thighs.

Please refer to Part III for the tables describing estrogen/progestin combinations (Table 20-f); estrogen/androgen combinations (Table 20-g); progesterone (Table 20-h); and progestins (Table 20-i).

Starting Hormone Replacement Therapy

Before starting HRT, a woman should talk about her medical history with her health-care provider, who should look for anything that may possibly contraindicate estrogen therapy.

Before I begin a patient on HRT, I complete a comprehensive health and family history. Even my long-term patients undergo this process because there may have been new health developments among family members that need to be considered. A complete physical exam is also performed, which includes a breast and pelvic exam. I also like to have a recent mammogram. I order a blood chemistry panel, which includes a lipid and liver profile, and a urinalysis.

You may begin HRT as soon as you are menopausal. For some perimenopausal women with severe symptoms, I prescribe a low dose of estrogen. As soon as they become menopausal, I may switch them to a higher dose depending upon their symptoms. If they still have a uterus, I will also add a progestin or a progesterone.

In the case of surgical menopause, I give the woman either a patch or an injection of estradiol before she leaves the hospital.

Finding the Right Dose for You

For short-term therapy to relieve symptoms, you should work with your health-care provider, and in some cases your compounding pharmacist, to find the right dose for you. If you want to get rid of menopausal symptoms, start with the lowest dose until your symptoms have resolved.

Women with premature menopause usually require a higher dose of estrogen. The younger they are, the higher the estrogen level their body is accustomed to. However, the level should be gradually decreased as they approach 50, since the risk of breast cancer is related to a higher dose of estrogen.[7]

Most women respond very well to the average dose of estrogen, 0.625 mg of Premarin, Tri-est 2.5 mg, Estrace 1 mg, Ogen 0.625 mg, Estratab 0.3 mg, or a .05 transdermal patch. Few women will need a higher dose. It has been my experience that a woman needs more estrogen when she is experiencing stress. Instead of increasing the estrogen level, I would rather add some testosterone or suggest a low dose of DHEA, 5 to 10 mg twice a day.

There are no long-term outcome studies on women who have had *physiological* replacement doses of estrogen. Until they are available for long-term therapy, when taken for the prevention of heart disease and osteoporosis, you should stick to the dosages that have been found to be therapeutic.

When Should Estrogen Therapy Cease?

Many health-care providers advocate the use of estrogen because of its multiple advantages. My belief is that if your symptoms are not responsive to alternative treatments, estrogen may be an appropriate alternative. However, I advise that after two to three years of estrogen therapy, consider tapering off after reevaluating your response and any potential personal risks. Prolonged use for *prevention of disease* should be carefully evaluated, and a decision needs to be made according to a woman's personal risk. (See chapter 20 for further reference: "Making the Right Decisions.")

Tapering Hormone Therapy

For a woman who has been on hormone therapy for more than a year, stopping it abruptly can wreak havoc. Some of my patients have complained of an acute recurrence of hot flashes, extreme depression, an inability to sleep or concentrate, and other symptoms. Except when estrogen has to be discontinued because of breast cancer, estrogen therapy should be stopped gradually, over a period of several weeks or months, depending on the duration of the therapy.

HRT benefits to the heart persist for several years after you stop, but disappear after ten years.

My patient, Bobbie, had been on Estrace for eight years when her older sister developed breast cancer. Bobbie decided to stop. The following regimen worked beautifully for her: She took Estrace Mondays through Fridays and took the weekend off for two months. For the next three-month period, she took Estrace every other day; during the next three months, she took it on Mondays and Thursdays, then once a week for three months, and then she finally stopped. If a patient starts having any symptoms, I usually advise her to return to the previous regimen until her symptoms have resolved for two to three months, then continue the tapering schedule.

Women who are on transdermal therapy may gradually cut their patch into smaller pieces and seal the patch with adhesive tape. However, it may be difficult to keep the patch from falling off. Some women may have an allergic reaction to the tape. Switching to an oral dose, then tapering off, may be a better solution.

You need to remember that after stopping HRT, over the subsequent few years there is rapid bone loss, just as would have happened after menopause, producing an increased risk of osteoporosis and hip fracture.

Follow-Up for Women on Estrogen Therapy

I continue to give a complete exam once a year to my patients who are on HRT, including a Pap smear, if appropriate. Their serum lipid profile is also monitored. I may order a bone density measurement, especially among women who are still smoking in spite of my badgering them! About 15 percent of smokers will develop osteoporosis, even though they are taking HRT. A mammogram is also done annually. I take advantage of each visit to review the reasons why the patient is taking HRT. Together we make the decision to continue or stop, depending upon her risk factors. I always recommend lifestyle habits that promote overall health and well-being.

Selective Estrogen Receptor Modulators (SERMs)

The estrogen debate would be moot if designer estrogens could be manufactured. These estrogens would be selective to the bone and brain, but spare the uterus and breast. SERMs mimic estrogen in some parts of the body, while acting against it in other parts.

Tamoxifen and Raloxifene are the most studied SERMs; there are many more to follow.

Tamoxifen: Studies have revealed that Tamoxifen also lowers the risk of breast cancer in high-risk women, as well as the risk of cardiovascular disease. (Please see chapter 8: "Breast Cancer: A Woman's Worst Fear.") The side effects of Tamoxifen include blood clots and an increased risk of uterine cancer.

Raloxifene: Raloxifene is approved for the prevention of osteoporosis. However, the media has been using "prevention" and "treatment" indiscriminately, which can be very confusing. Raloxifene has no effect on hot flashes, mood swings, or thinning of vaginal tissues. The most common side effect of Raloxifene is hot flashes and leg cramps. A rare, but serious, side effect of Raloxifene is an increased risk of blood clots.

Studies with Raloxifene reveal promising outcomes on lipid profiles. Raloxifene decreases total cholesterol and LDL but has no effect on HDL. Studies have suggested that HDL is the best predictor of coronary heart disease risk in women, and that up to half of the apparent cardiovascular benefit observed in estrogen-treated women may be mediated by the higher HDL levels. The question remains: Will the use of Raloxifene translate in decreasing the risk of heart disease?

If Raloxifene increases bone density, does it also prevent fractures? It has a positive effect on lipid profiles: Does it also prevent heart attacks? A large ongoing study by pharmaceutical giant Eli Lilly, with 77,000 women aged 60 to 75 in more than 20 countries, is looking at the rate of spine fracture, breast cancer, mental acuity, heart attack, stroke, and other side effects.

It is important to keep in mind that all of the SERMs that are coming onto the market have only been studied for a short period of time. No one knows the long-term effects of these drugs. Ongoing studies will help. The lesson here is that women should wait until more data is available.

℀ ℀ ℀

You are probably still confused about whether you should use HRT or try an alternative approach—well, you are not alone! (For more information, see chapter 20: "Making the Right Decisions for You.")

CHAPTER 6

Cardiovascular Disease (CVD) and Women

According to a recent telephone survey published in the *Journal of Woman's Health,* women remain unaware of their risks of cardiovascular disease (CVD). The journal reported that 745 respondents rated themselves as knowledgeable about women's health issues; however, 34 percent thought that they were more likely to die of breast cancer than CVD. The fact is that every year, 250,000 deaths are caused by CVD, versus 44,000 caused by breast cancer, 6,000 caused by endometrial cancer, and 135,000 caused by other types of cancer.

Facts about CVD

- One out of every two women dies each year of heart disease.

- Since 1984, CVD-associated mortality for women has surpassed that for men.[1]

- One in nine women experiences some form of CVD between the ages of 45 and 64.

- One in three women experiences some form of CVD after age 65.

- About 250,000 women die from a heart attack each year.

- If a woman has a heart attack, she is twice as likely as a man to die within the first few weeks.

- More women than men die during the first year after a heart attack.[2]

- Black women have a 22 percent greater risk of heart attack, and 75 percent greater risk of stroke, than white women. Black women are more likely to die from heart disease than white women. Mexican-American and African-American women face a greater risk of cardiovascular disease than white women do. There is a higher incidence of CVD among black and Mexican-American women than among white women of comparable socioeconomic status.[3] The discrepancy appears to be associated with cost barriers, unavailability of health insurance, and discrimination in health care.[4]

The most common risk factors for cardiovascular disease are the following:

- Age: The older you are, the greater your risk. With age, blood vessels become narrower and less flexible.

- Family history: You are at greater risk if your mother had a heart attack before age 65, or your father before age 55.

- Smoking, which accounts for one-fifth of CVD deaths.

- Cholesterol levels: Increased total cholesterol, increased levels of low density lipoprotein (LDL) cholesterol greater than 130, low levels (less than 35) of high density lipoprotein (HDL), and triglyceride levels of greater than 400 mg/dL increase the risk for CVD. With high cholesterol, there is a fatty deposit, or plaque, in blood vessels.

- People with hypertension or diabetes; and those who lead a sedentary lifestyle and are obese, are also at a greater risk of CVD.

- Stress: A relationship between stress and CVD has been established. The belief is that stress increases heart rate and blood pressure.

Cholesterol and Cardiovascular Disease

More than 50 million women have elevated total cholesterol. When cholesterol in the bloodstream is high, it sticks to the inside walls of the blood vessels, narrowing them, and sometimes blocking them entirely. Cholesterol settles in the coronary arteries, endangering the heart. When cholesterol builds up in the arteries of the neck, it increases the risk of stroke and endangers the brain.

Types of cholesterol: Cholesterol is a type of fat manufactured in the body, mostly by the liver and the intestines, and it is found in every cell in the body. Cholesterol is necessary to support vital functions, such as the synthesis of cell membranes, nerve insulation, sex hormone production, and production of bile for the digestive system.

The body produces about two-thirds of the blood cholesterol needed; the other one-third comes from the food we eat.

Cholesterol travels through the blood in packages, called lipoproteins. Lipoproteins are classified by the basis of the protein content. They can be HDL (high-density lipoprotein), LDL (low-density lipoprotein), and VLDL (very low-density lipoprotein). LDL, or "bad cholesterol," is responsible for the buildup of fat in the artery walls and the formation of plaque. Arteries that are damaged by LDL attract white blood cells, form a plaque that hardens, and causes a narrowing of arteries, thus producing angina. HDL, or "good cholesterol," sweeps up the debris left by LDL, and carries it back into the liver to be broken down.

Triglycerides are another fat found in the bloodstream. Lipoproteins, which are rich in triglycerides, also contain cholesterol-producing atherosclerosis. When triglyceride levels are high, this potentiates the negative effects of LDL to cause lesions in the blood vessels.

Your cholesterol levels are affected by heredity, diet, weight, degree of physical activity, age, sex, and alcohol consumption. Cholesterol is also found in animal-derived food sources, including meat, eggs, and dairy products.

Table 6-a
CHECKING YOUR LIPID PROFILE LEVELS
< = Less than   > = More than

	Good	Borderline	Bad
Total Cholesterol	<200	200–239	>240
HDL	>60	35–69	<35
LDL	<130	130–159	>160
Triglycerides	50–200	200-500	>500

You should begin regular cholesterol testing by age 20. Fasting is not necessary, but total and HDL cholesterol levels should be measured. If the total cholesterol level is greater than 200, or HDL cholesterol is less than 35, you will need to fast for 9 to 12 hours and obtain a lipid profile, which indicates total cholesterol, HDL, triglycerides, and estimated LDL cholesterol levels.

An elevated LDL to HDL ratio is another indicator of CVD. The ratio should not be greater than 4:1.

Controlling High Cholesterol

Lifestyle modification, dietary therapy, weight control, and exercise should be the first approaches to lowering lipid levels. Lipid levels tests should be repeated after following a low-cholesterol diet for three months. If levels remain high, you should go on a much stricter diet where your cholesterol intake must be less than 200 mg/day, and saturated fat should be limited to less than 7 percent of daily calories. You may need the help of a nutritionist with this diet.

A weight-reduction program should be initiated in combination with dietary therapy to reduce cholesterol levels. Weight reduction also raises HDL levels, and reduces triglyceride levels and blood pressure.

Many studies have shown that moderate exercise, several times a week, helps raise HDL and lower LDL in women. (See chapter 14: "If You're

Sedentary, Learn to Exercise.") When combined with a low-fat, low-calorie diet, the results are even better.

If you are postmenopausal and have tried all of the above for more than six months and your lipid values are still elevated, you and your health-care provider should consider drug therapy. Women with known clinical heart disease who take a cholesterol-lowering drug can reduce their mortality up to 24 percent.

Before starting drug therapy, two lipid profiles should be obtained at one-month intervals. Drug therapy is not usually recommended before the onset of menopause in women who have no other risks for CVD, because of the side effects, cost, and inconvenience. Treatment is reserved only for those women with an LDL greater than 220 mg/dL.

For postmenopausal women, 55 years and older, without CVD, drug therapy is recommended for LDL greater than 190, with no or one risk factor(s) for CVD. If a woman has two or more risk factors and an LDL greater than 160, she should be treated with drug therapy.

A lipid profile should be obtained six to eight weeks following the initiation of drug therapy, and again six weeks later. When the profile is within the target range, it should be repeated every three to four months for a year, then every four to six months thereafter.

Estrogen replacement therapy and high cholesterol: Studies have revealed that estrogen reduces LDL-cholesterol by 15 percent, and increases HDL-cholesterol levels up to 15 percent; however, estrogen has been shown to increase triglyceride levels.

Stress and cardiovascular disease: A study published in *JAMA* confirmed that mental stress does increase the risk of myocardial death.

Homocysteine and cardiovascular disease: One-fourth of all heart attacks occur among people with no known risk factors. New studies suggest that homocysteine, an amino acid derived from dietary protein, plays a critical role in causing injury to the walls of arteries—a role as injurious as smoking. [5]

Homocysteine levels have not been fully accepted in the general medical community as a major risk factor for heart disease. Generally, homocysteine level testing is reserved for young patients without clear-cut reasons for CVD. Those with elevated homocysteine are treated with 1 mg of folic acid per day.

Other etiologies may include cytomegalovirus infection, chlamydia, pneumonia, and *porphyromanas gingivalis*, which causes gum inflammation.

Minimizing Your Risk of Developing Cardiovascular Disease

You cannot control whether you are a woman, are black, or have a family history of heart disease. But there are factors that you *can* control, some of which are listed below.

By implementing a healthy diet and lifestyle, 95 percent of heart disease can be prevented. (A study published in *JAMA* confirmed that mental stress does increase the risk of myocardial death.)

Smoking: An estimated 30 percent of deaths from heart disease are attributable to smoking. Prevention of the underlying disease process, arteriosclerosis (hardening of the arteries), is imperative. Smoking cessation is associated with a 50 to 70 percent reduction in the risk of cardiovascular disease. The risk of cardiovascular disease among ex-smokers is reduced to nearly half that of smokers. (See chapter 15: "If You Smoke, You Must Quit.")

Hypertension: Hypertension, or high blood pressure, is known as the "silent killer," and is a significant risk factor for CVD.[6]

Blood pressure is considered normal between 120 mm Hg systolic, and 80 mm Hg diastolic. If the systolic is higher than 140, and the diastolic is higher than 90, it is considered high blood pressure.

— *Blood pressure measurement*: The Sixth Report of the Joint National Committee on Detection, Evaluation and Treatment of High Blood Pressure (JNC VI), which was published in November 1997, established a blood pressure classification for adults, age 18 and older.

Table 6-b

BLOOD PRESSURE FOR ADULTS AGE 18 YEARS AND OLDER

Category	Systolic mmHg		Diastolic mmHg
Optimal	<120	and	<80
Normal	<130	and	<85
High Normal	130–139	and/or	85–89

Table 6-c

HYPERTENSION

	Systolic	Diastolic
Normal blood pressure	<140	<90
Mild hypertension	140–159	90–99
Moderate hypertension	160–179	100–109
Severe hypertension	180–209	110–119
Very severe hypertension	>209	>119

Treatment for hypertension should not be initiated unless your blood pressure is very high—more than 200/100. Treatment should only be used after conservative approaches such as losing weight, establishing a regular exercise program, yoga, meditation, stress reduction, biofeedback, and herbs have failed.

Cardiovascular Disease and . . .

. . . **Diabetes:** Women with diabetes have twice the risk of developing heart attacks as nondiabetic women. Keeping your weight under control is a good way to prevent diabetes. Almost 80 percent of diabetics are obese. Obesity is one of the most preventable underlying risk factors for Type 2 diabetes. Losing 10 to 15 percent of body weight reduces all of the risks associated with obesity. A diet low in fat, high in fibers, and with lots of fruits and vegetables has been associated with a decreased risk of cancer, heart disease, diabetes, and stroke.

. . . **Obesity:** People who are obese eat more calories than they need; they also have bad eating habits that can contribute to high cholesterol levels. People who are obese have an increased risk of heart disease.[6] They also tend to have a higher-than-normal risk of high blood pressure, diabetes, and gallstones.

. . . **Diet:** Eating a proper diet can significantly reduce your risk of CVD. Coronary heart disease among women is more closely related to the type of fat consumed than total fat intake, according to one study, which concluded that replacing saturated and trans-unsaturated fats with unhydrogenated mono-unsaturated and polyunsaturated fat is more effective in preventing coronary heart disease among women than reducing overall fat intake.

. . . **Exercise:** Regular exercise plays a major role in preventing heart disease. Women who lead a sedentary lifestyle are three times more likely to die from a heart attack than active women. Regular exercise has been demonstrated to reduce the risk of CVD by 45 percent. Vigorous exercise reduces the risk of a heart attack by half.

. . . **Estrogen:** Disease-causing, blocked blood vessels are less common among women younger than age 55 than among men younger than age 55, but this difference decreases with age. By age 80, the rates are equal for men and women.

After menopause, total cholesterol, triglycerides, and LDL increase, while HDL decreases. There is also an increase in fibrinogen, which is a risk factor for CVD and strokes. Many studies have revealed that women who take estrogen for several years after menopause experience a 35 to 50 percent lower risk of CVD. Estrogen decreases atherosclerotic plaque size by 50 percent, possibly by lowering LDL and fibrinogen. Estrogen has been documented to decrease LDL by 15 percent. Estrogen increases HDL, but also increases triglycerides. The cardio-protective effect of estrogen is strongest among current users. The benefit diminishes three years after estrogen cessation.

. . . **Aspirin:** To prevent heart disease, perimenopausal and menopausal women can take one baby aspirin each day, unless there is a contraindication for using aspirin. Also remember that before taking any long-term medications, including aspirin, you should consult your health-care provider. Aspirin has been found to reduce the risk of a second heart attack among women. It may also help prevent a first heart attack.

. . . **Traditional Chinese medicine:** According to traditional Chinese medicine, heart disease is caused by heart weakness, blocked energy flow, and poor digestion, resulting in the buildup of plaque in the arteries. To strengthen the digestive system, herbs and acupuncture are recommended.

. . . **Ayurvedic medicine:** Ayurvedic doctors use diet, purification techniques, and detoxification to remove free radicals that cause heart disease.

REDUCE YOUR RISK OF CARDIOVASCULAR DISEASE

- Keep your blood pressure, diabetes, lipid levels, and weight under control
- Use HRT
- Engage in stress-management techniques
- Eat healthful foods and supplements
- Exercise regularly
- Stop smoking
- Use alcohol in moderation
- Practice mind-body interventions
- Take baby aspirin

To assess your risk of heart disease, please refer to Questionnaire I in chapter 20.

CHAPTER 7

Osteoporosis

*O*steoporosis literally means "porous bone" or "bones with tiny holes." Due to the loss of bone density, the risk of fracture from trivial accidents is increased. Bone mass in women continues to increase early in life, and reaches maximum mass by age 35.

Peak bone mass is determined by genetic predisposition, nutrition, hormones, body mass, and weight-bearing exercise.[1] Of the nutritional factors, calcium has the greatest significance. Studies have shown that maximizing calcium intake during the growth years and up to age 30 or 35 greatly affects a woman's peak bone mass.

After the age of 35, a woman loses bone mass at a rate of one percent per year. Men also lose bone, but at a lesser rate, because testosterone protects bone.

Age-related bone loss is normal. The rate of bone loss usually accelerates after menopause, sometimes dramatically, because of the decrease in the production of estrogen, which plays an important part in maintaining bone density. Whether or not you develop osteoporosis will depend on how much bone mass you had when you began menopause, and how quickly it is lost.

Approximately 25 million American women suffer from osteoporosis. Osteoporosis also contributes to approximately 1.5 million bone fractures per year, with an estimated treatment cost of over $10 billion!

Vertebral deformity is the most frequent manifestation of osteoporosis, clinically seen as a loss of height and pronounced curvature of the spine. Vertebral crush fractures occur when one vertebra collapses. When this happens to multiple vertebrae, it can cause back pain, the loss of height, and a hunched-over appearance; in extreme cases a "dowager's hump" may result. Colles' fractures, which occur in the bones of the wrist and forearm, happen during a fall and can also be due to osteoporosis. Hip fracture is the most severe consequence of osteoporosis.

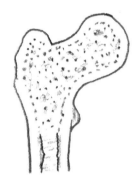
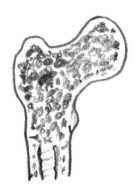

Figure 7-a: Normal bone   **Figure 7-b: Osteoporotic bone**

Osteoporosis and Black Women

Women of African descent have a bone density that is 20 times higher than European women. The reason is not well understood.

Black women are still at risk for osteoporosis even though the incidence is much lower than for white women. Bone loss may occur later in life for black women, but this loss can progress twice as fast as for white women of the same age. Black women have less risk of hip fractures than white women.[2] By age 70, bone loss accelerates in black women, and by age 75, the incidence of hip fractures among black women is almost the same when compared to white women.

Risk Factors for Osteoporosis

The precise cause of osteoporosis is unknown; estrogen deficiency is acknowledged as a major cause of postmenopausal osteoporosis, and many studies show that inactivity and calcium deficiency are some precipitating factors. Many endocrine conditions, such as hyperthyroidism (overactive thyroid); Cushing syndrome (overactive secretions of the adrenal gland); hyperparathyroidism (overactive parathyroid glands); steroids; thyroid hormones; anticonvulsives; anticoagulants; antacids that contains aluminum; some diuretics; eating disorders; cigarette smoking and alcohol abuse; and Tamoxifen (premenopausal use)—all contribute to bone loss and may be related to the development of osteoporosis.

Perimenopausal women who lack menstrual periods, including those with low estrogen, marathon runners, gymnasts, and athletes are also at risk of developing osteoporosis.[3]

Alcohol abuse causes a direct change in bone cells. It also causes liver impairment and problems metabolizing vitamin D. Drunkenness will increase the risk of falling. Alcoholics usually have poor dietary habits.

According to the Framingham study, there may be an association between an increased risk of hip fracture and consumption of more than two and a half cups of caffeine per day.

Diagnosis of Osteoporosis

It is best to diagnose osteoporosis in its early stages, before bone fractures occur. To determine this, a bone mineral density (BMD) test is required. To understand the test, a T-Score represents the number of standard deviations between a given bone density and the density of a normal 35-year-old white woman.

The World Health Organization defines osteoporosis in white women as more than 2.5 standard deviations (level of changes) from normal. Osteopenia, or low bone mass, is defined as one standard deviation from normal.

Bone mineral density (BMD) measurement: Bone mineral density is a simple, painless way to diagnose osteoporosis. This test determines the thickness of the bone, using a small amount of radiation or ultrasound. It only takes a few minutes, with one-tenth the radiation of a standard chest x-ray.

Hip measurements can only be obtained with dual-energy x-ray absorptiometry (DEXA) scanners, and they are not readily available.

HOW THE BONE MINERAL
DENSITY TEST IS INTERPRETED

T-Score	Meaning
+ 1 to -1	Normal
-1 to -2.5	Slightly low; you have slight bone loss that may indicate osteopenia
-2.5 and below	You have bone loss that may indicate osteoporosis

---

For every one point decrease in the level of bone mineral density, there is a 2.6-times increased risk of fracture.

Can bone mineral density at menopause really predict what will happen around age 70 when most fractures occur? More studies are necessary to answer this question.

Who should have a bone mineral density test? The BMD test is not recommended for healthy perimenopausal women. Screening should be reserved for high-risk perimenopausal women and only be ordered if the result is going to influence a decision. Women at high risk are those with an x-ray suggestive of osteopenia, women receiving long-term steroid therapy, those with a history of eating disorders such as anorexia nervosa, and women diagnosed with primary asymptomatic hyperparathyroidism.

BMD may be performed after menopause for non-black women who have decided not to go on HRT.

After menopause, you should have a BMD:

- if you are a black woman 55 years or older and have never been on HRT. You should have a baseline BMD and repeat it every two to three years. If you are 60 years or older and have been on HRT, or have decided not to continue with HRT, you may want to have a baseline BMD and repeat it every two to three years. Up to 15 percent of women on HRT can still develop osteoporosis.

- if you are a postmenopausal Caucasian, Asian, Hispanic, or Native American and have never been on HRT. You should have a baseline BMD and repeat it every two to three years. If you are 60 years or older and have been on HRT, or have decided not to continue with HRT, you may want to have a baseline BMD and repeat it every two to three years.

Also, according to the National Osteoporosis Foundation in collaboration with nine other medical organizations, all white women over the age of 65 should have a BMD test.

In cases of osteopenia, after one to two years treatment, a BMD is then repeated. In cases of osteoporosis, after one to two years of treatment, a BMD is then repeated. A BMD test has a 2 to 3 percent margin of error.

Bone mineral density testing: There are several kind of tests, all involving x-rays. The DEXA for the whole body is the "gold standard" for hip fracture prevention. The Acu-DEXA, for the fingers, has become more readily available.

Quantitative ultrasound: Ultrasound does not measure bone density, but measures values that predict fractures independent of BMD.

Your foot is inserted into a small box about the size of a laser printer. Bone density is determined by how easily and quickly the sound waves penetrate the bones. The result can be printed out for you. The test generally costs about $40; the typical cost of an x-ray is $127.

Biochemical markers: The rate of bone loss (resorption) and bone formation can be assessed by measuring specific markers. They are mostly used to see if a treatment is working. A 30 percent reduction in a marker's level means that a particular treatment is working.

Prevention of Osteoporosis

Osteoporosis can and should be prevented. Once bone mass is lost, it is almost impossible to replace it.

Diet and osteoporosis: Many vitamins and minerals are involved in the prevention and treatment of osteoporosis—not just calcium. Bones are made from calcium phosphate, calcium carbonate, magnesium, fluoride, and other minerals. Healthy bone needs minerals such as calcium, magnesium, manganese, zinc, boron, silicone, copper, and stronton. In a 1990 study, broad-spectrum vitamins and minerals, a healthy diet, and adequate hormone levels were attributed to an 11 percent increase in bone density over a one-year period.

Too much calcium can also be detrimental to the absorption of other minerals. One study revealed that calcium can interfere with the absorption of iron, magnesium, and possibly zinc.

Calcium and osteoporosis: See chapter 12: "Calcium and Your Health."

Exercise and osteoporosis: Exercise increases bone density, while physical inactivity tends to cause thinning of the bone. This can be seen among individuals who are bedridden for a long time or among astronauts who stay in weightless conditions for extended periods.

Weight-bearing exercise, such as walking, dancing, bicycling, and jogging—prior to age 35—stimulates bone cells to grow and leads to an increase in bone mass.

High-intensity resistance training (using weights) also increases bone density and muscle mass, and age is no barrier.[4] Other exercises that help prevent osteoporosis are running, aerobics, cross-country skiing, stair climbing, and tennis. The optimal type and amount of physical activity to prevent osteoporosis has not been established.

A study on bone mineral density in mothers and daughters revealed that in cases where the mother had osteoporosis, the daughter could reduce her risk of osteoporosis and increase her bone density with regular exercise and calcium supplementation.

Phytoestrogens and osteoporosis: There are ongoing human studies to determine whether phytoestrogens can prevent osteoporosis. In a study performed with monkeys, soy phytoestrogens failed to maintain bone density. Another study revealed that soy foods increased bone density after six months. In rats, soy protein does not result in urine calcium loss; it reduces femoral and vertebral bone loss and suppresses osteoblast activity.

When Should Treatment Be Initiated?

As with any treatment, there are always risks and benefits involved. The first recommendation should be a regimen of calcium and vitamin D supplementation, a nutritious diet, and exercise, followed by a bone density test two years later. Bone markers can be measured in six months to see if the regimen is working. It takes at least two years to see a change in bone mineral density. Prescription drugs should be added only when conservative treatments are not working. In some cases, prescription drugs may be used in conjunction with a conservative approach when there is strong evidence that the benefit of using prescription drugs outweighs any potential risks. It should also show that using prescription drugs would effectively prevent fractures and their consequences.

Drugs for the Prevention of Osteoporosis

Estrogen replacement therapy (ERT): Estrogen is indicated for the prevention of osteoporosis, as it inhibits bone resorption and decreases the risk of osteoporosis; however, it does not eliminate it. ERT, CEE 0.625 mg or equivalent, maintains bone in about 85 percent of postmenopausal women.[5] There is also a 60 percent decrease in spinal fractures and a 25 percent decrease in other fractures with five years of estrogen replacement therapy.

ERT does not stem bone loss in all women, especially smokers. Approximately 15 percent of female smokers who are on ERT may have osteoporosis.

According to the PEPI trial, older women with low initial bone mineral density and those with no previous hormone use gained bone mass at clinically important sites in the body.

The ideal minimum dose of estrogen for preventing and reducing bone loss has yet to be established, but lower doses, with fewer side effects, are better than no estrogen at all. The majority of studies that support the premise that estrogen prevents osteoporosis were done with Premarin 0.625 mg. Taking Premarin 0.3 mg with 1,500 mg of calcium had the same level of bone protection compared to those who took 0.625 mg.[6]

In a two-year double-blind placebo-controlled, randomized study conducted with 406 postmenopausal women, Estratab 0.3 mg was demonstrated to be effective in the prevention of postmenopausal osteoporosis when compared to a placebo. There was only one case of endometrial hyperplasia in the groups treated with a placebo and Estratab tablets.

The Rancho Bernardo Study, published in 1997, concluded that estrogen initiated in the menopausal period and continued into late life was associated with the highest bone density. Nevertheless, estrogen when begun after age 60, appears to offer nearly an equal bone-conserving benefit.[7] After estrogen is stopped, bone loss starts again. Estrogen therapy only delays bone loss.

It has been suggested that since a woman's lifetime risk of osteoporosis and heart disease is greatly determined by her risks after age 65, using strategies such as taking HRT for five years, stopping it, and then restarting it after age 60 or 65 could also reduce her risk of fractures and heart disease, while not increasing her risk for breast cancer.

Biophosphonates and osteoporosis prevention: Alendronate (Fosamax) 5 mg, has been approved for the prevention of osteoporosis in postmenopausal women. Women with low bone mass and early menopause taking 5 mg for three years recognized an increase of 3.4 percent in spinal bone mineral density and an increase of 1.8 percent in the hip.

In a two-year study comparing Alendronate 5 mg with HRT (conjugated estrogen, CEE 0.625 mg and MPA 5 mg), there were equivalent increases in the BMD of the spine and hip. Alendronate, when given for three years, increases the average BMD about 9 percent in the spine and 6 percent over the femoral neck. New vertebral fractures were reduced by 48 percent. Alendronate may provide some long-term effects even after treatment has stopped. It stays on the bone for 10 to 12 years.

The failure rate of Alendronate 5 mg to prevent osteoporosis is 15 percent; however, Alendronate 10 mg produces twice the bone benefit that Raloxifene does.

Side effects of Alendronate may include abdominal and musculoskeletal pain, nausea, heart burn, constipation, diarrhea, and in rare cases, esophageal ulcers. When taken as directed, these side effects are the same as those of women in a placebo group. It should be taken with six to eight ounces of water, first thing in the morning; you should remain upright and not eat or drink anything for 30 minutes.

Alendronate is contraindicated in women with abnormalities of the esophagus, and those with the inability to stand or sit upright for at least 30 minutes.

Calcium supplements and antacids can interfere with the absorption of alendronate and should be taken at least a half hour later.

The duration of use of biophosphonates is only recommended for three to four years.

Raloxifene and osteoporosis: Raloxifene is not as effective as estrogen in preventing osteoporosis. It has been shown to reduce spinal fractures by 50 percent. Raloxifene is administered in a single daily dose of 60 mg and may be given without regard to meals or time of day.

Progesterone and osteoporosis: According to Jerilynn C. Prior, M.D., of the Division of Endocrinology and Metabolism at the University of British Columbia in Vancouver, there is evidence that progesterone stimulates bone formation. John Lee, M.D., is also a proponent of progesterone therapy for osteoporosis.

Androgens and osteoporosis: One study showed that a combination of estrogen and androgens may build bone mass more effectively than estrogen alone.[8]

Hip Fractures and Osteoporosis

Every year, women in the United States suffer at least 600,000 bone fractures directly caused by osteoporosis. Approximately 250,000 persons are hospitalized each year as a result of hip fracture, at a cost of $8.7 billion. Eighty-five percent of these were people over age 65. Five percent die in the hospital. About 50 percent of these people are discharged to nursing homes; half of those remain there. Less than 30 percent regain their previous functional level. More than 90 percent of hip fractures occur among women older than age 70; the average age is 80.

Having a normal bone density does not preclude you from suffering a hip fracture. Women with high or moderate bone density can still have fractures, accounting for a greater proportion of fractures among women. Being Asian has been classified as a risk factor for osteoporosis because of low bone mass; however, Asian women have less incidence of hip fractures than white women.

Risks factors for fractures: According to an ongoing cohort study and the Study of Osteoporotic Fractures Research Group (SOF),[9] the various risk factors that lead to fractures are a complex interaction including low bone density, frailty, weakness, and the likelihood of falling. The thin, frail, and elderly have more of a tendency to fall, resulting in a fracture because of a lack of padding; elderly females are more likely to be taking sleeping pills and psychotropic drugs, which alter balance.

Reducing your fracture risk: A recent study revealed that diet alone can have a positive effect in reducing fractures. A dietary combination of vitamin D and calcium moderately reduced bone loss in the femoral neck, spine, and total body over three years, and reduced the incidence of non-vertebral fractures.

Preventing falls: Many osteoporosis patients are at risk for fracture, but falling is more directly related to fracturing of the hip. The likelihood of falling increases exponentially with age. Drugs may cause dizziness or disorientation and can contribute to falling. Changes in gait, mobility, and risk of falls increases with medication, which can cause hypotension, central nervous system depression, or movement disorders. Caution should be taken to prevent falls.

You need to learn how to live safely and to prevent falls and other injuries:

- Maintain proper lighting around the house, especially in stair areas.
- Do not let toys or small objects remain on the floor; keep hallways uncluttered.
- Avoid loose carpeting; do not put throw rugs at the top or bottom of stairs.
- In the kitchen, place a rubber mat near the sink and wear rubber-soled shoes.
- Clean up spills on flooring immediately.
- On the shower floor or tub, put a nonskid adhesive strip or a rubber mat; add a shower seat and grab bars.
- Use handrails when going up and down stairs.

- Arrange furniture so you can move from one place to another with ease.
- Keep telephones and electrical cords out of walking paths.

Treatment of Osteoporosis

Treatment of osteoporosis consists of estrogen replacement therapy, Alendronate 10 mg, and calcitonin, which have been demonstrated to increase bone density and decrease vertebral fracture risk and height loss.[10] Calcitonin has been shown to reduce the risk of spinal fracture by 35 to 45 percent. Calcitonin is a naturally occurring hormone produced by the thyroid gland. Calcitonin is recommended for women who are at least five years into menopause.

Calcitonin-salmon (Miacalcin Nasal Spray)—one puff a day of 200 IU—and calcitonin injectable, slow further bone loss and may increase bone density in some women. Calcitonin spray reduces spinal fracture and decreases pain from recent spinal compression fractures among 50 percent of women. There are no long-term side effects. Injectable calcitonin is reserved for women with severe osteoporosis and preexisting vertebral fractures. It decreases the risk of new vertebral fractures by 75 percent. Calcitonin also reduces the pain associated with symptomatic vertebral fractures.

Alendronate, when given 10 mg a day together with 500 to 1,000 mg of calcium after three years, showed an increase of bone mineral density by 8 percent, and a reduction in the risk of fracture by 50 percent.

An article in *JAMA* documented an additive effect on bone density among women who were given 10 mg of alendronate and who were not responding to estrogen replacement therapy.

Sodium fluoride is the only available drug with new bone formation. It is reserved for those with severe osteoporosis (BMD <4).

BONE HEALTH MADE EASY

(A quick summary on how to maintain bone health)

- Use stress-management techniques
- Eat healthfully; take calcium, vitamin D, and minerals
- Exercise with weights
- Stop smoking
- Use alcohol, caffeine, and soft drinks in moderation
- Familiarize yourself with fracture-prevention strategies

To assess your risk for osteoporosis, please refer to Questionnaire II in chapter 20.

CHAPTER 8

Breast Cancer: A Woman's Worst Fear

The Female Breast

The female breast is an important element of a woman's sexuality. The breast consists of mammary glands, which are capable of producing milk. These glands empty into a system of ducts that lead to the nipple. These glands and ducts are surrounded by fatty tissue. The breast tissue extends into the armpit, where lymph nodes are present. Lymph nodes are bean-shaped structures that are scattered along the vessels of the lymph system. The nodes act as filters, collecting bacteria or cancer cells that may travel through the system. The size of a woman's breast is determined by her genes (if not her plastic surgeon).

A PERSONAL STORY

My relationship with my breasts started on the wrong foot. I was a tomboy born to a 5'8" father and a 4'9" mother. For whatever reason, I was destined to be six feet tall in a country where the average woman was about 5'2". I was the firstborn. My sister Marise, who is now 5'4", had breasts by age

10 and was menstruating by age 12. Like everything else that I do in my life, I had to be different. While my little sister was becoming a woman in front of my eyes, I was growing taller and taller, with no sign of puberty.

I don't mean to shock you, but I grew up thinking I wanted to be a man, because in my society they had everything! When Grandma heard me say such drastic things, she tried to talk some sense into me. She got on her knees and asked God to forgive me, then explained to me that I could still be a woman and have everything I wanted. I liked the explanation, but not the fact that I had to see a doctor because I was not menstruating yet. And the notion of possibly having to take medication was even more undesirable.

But, I did go. The male doctor took a look at my naked, lanky body and decided that nothing was wrong with me. I was just going through a growth spurt and eventually would have body hair, breasts, and then periods. He also told Grandma that she had to fatten me up, that I did not have sufficient body fat to make those dreadful "things" happen. When I found out that "being a woman" meant menstruating for another 35 years, I was not a happy girl.

When breasts finally appeared, I was 14 years old. I never undressed in front of Marise or anyone else. I was too ashamed to be seen naked. It was not until a trip to New York, years later, that Marise and my other sister, Elsie, locked the bedroom door and told me that they would not let me out until I let them take a peek at my breasts. I looked into their eyes; they were serious. So I flashed them and ran.

My breasts were always "in the way," something that grew out of my body that I could care less about. The uncomfortable relationship with my breasts finally changed when I went to one of Dr. Christiane Northrup's lectures (where I met Louise Hay). Christiane mentioned that we have to love every part of our bodies; if we do not, then something might happen to get rid of it.

After I read Louise's book *Heal Your Body,* the relationship with my breasts definitely changed for the better. Now, when I look at them, I see that they are gorgeous and still hanging in there: I see them as a part of myself. They have been with me now for over 30 years, are an essential part of my femininity, and have brought me many sensual pleasures. When I am naked in front of the mirror, I look at them, then cup them in my hands and tell them: "Not to worry, my friends, you are safe with me."

Breast Tenderness

My experience has been that when a patient complains of breast tenderness, with or without palpation, it is typically due to tenderness of the underlying chest-wall muscle. Often these women will confess that they had been moving furniture, lifting a grandchild, or had embarked on a new exercise routine with weight lifting. The pain usually resolves with rest, and occasionally, a mild analgesic.

Another potential cause of breast pain is excessive caffeine intake. Caffeine is present in many soft drinks and chocolate, in addition to coffee. Some analgesics may also contain caffeine. Abstaining from caffeine has proven to be very beneficial to women with breast pain.

Other causes of breast pain are fibrocystic changes worsened by premenstrual fluid retention; beginning hormone replacement therapy; cysts; injuries to the chest wall or to the nerves near the breast; or costochondritis, an inflammation of the breast bone.

Breast Cancer and Women

One out of nine women will develop breast cancer sometime in her life. Women with a family history of breast cancer have a two to ten times higher incidence of breast cancer than the general female population. In the United States, an estimated 175,000 women will be diagnosed with breast cancer in 1999. Of these, 43,300 will die of the disease. This type of cancer is more common in older women, but can strike women of any age. The average age at diagnosis is 62, with 25 percent of cancers in the breast being reported among women aged 40 to 50.

Monthly breast self-exams, regular exams from your health-care provider, and breast x-rays (mammograms) are the first line of defense. Very few women perform regular breast self-exams or have mammogram screenings as recommended.

Fortunately, 90 percent of breast cancers that are detected early—with a mammogram while they're too small to be felt—are curable, meaning that the woman lives for five or more additional years after treatment.

Many women are frightened by the incidence of breast cancer, so it's important to put it in perspective.

Deaths Due to Heart Disease	**Deaths Due to Breast Cancer**
1 in 2 per year	1 in 25 per year

The majority of breast tumors, about 80 percent, are benign or non-cancerous. A lump that is benign is highly unlikely to become cancerous. These include cysts, firm tumors called fibroadenomas, and fibrocystic changes that are associated with aging. Two-thirds of newly diagnosed breast cancers are localized—they have not spread to other parts of the body. This often means that the woman can choose a surgical procedure that removes only the cancer (a lumpectomy) rather than the entire breast (a mastectomy).

No one knows why women develop breast cancer or why the incidence is increasing. Perhaps the increase is due to the greater use of mammography screening, especially among young women, which reveals some cancers sooner. Another possibility is that women are simply living longer, allowing the development of cancer to finally catch up with them. The role of diet, drugs, and the environment in the development of breast cancer has not yet been determined. The breast cancer genes BRCA1 "breast cancer 1," gene prevalent in families with ovarian and breast cancer; and the BRCA2 "breast cancer 2" gene, prevalent in families with both male and female breast cancer, are only responsible for 5 to 10 percent of breast cancers.

Who Has an Increased Risk of Developing Breast Cancer?

The leading risk factors for breast cancer are simply being female and getting older. About 75 percent of women diagnosed with breast cancer have no identifiable risk factors. It has been suggested that if a woman's mother, sister, half-sister, or daughter has had breast cancer, she is at a higher-than-average risk of developing the disease. Other circumstances correlating with higher risk include being Caucasian, being older than 50 years of age, not having given birth to a child, and becoming a mother for the first time when over the age of 30.

Others at higher risk include women who started their period early or entered menopause very late (over the age of 55); very obese women, women with extra weight distributed in the upper body and stomach, rather than in the hips and thighs; women with a history of benign disease confirmed by biopsy; women with a high socioeconomic status; women on estrogen replacement therapy after menopause; women who have been on the Pill for a very long period; women with a specific genetic mutation, such as BRCA-1 and BRCA-2 genes, which increases susceptibility; and women with at least 75 percent of breast tissue so dense that interpretation of a mammogram is problematic.

Table 8-a
YOUR RISK OF GETTING BREAST CANCER

Age	Risk	Age	Risk
25	1 in 19,608	60	1 in 24
30	1 in 2,525	65	1 in 17
35	1 in 622	70	1 in 14
40	1 in 217	75	1 in 11
45	1 in 93	80	1 in 10
50	1 in 50	85	1 in 9
55	1 in 33	90	1 in 8
		95	1 in 8

Your risk may be slightly higher if you have a family history of breast cancer.

Facts about Black Women and Breast Cancer

Between 1988 and 1992, the most common cancers among blacks were lung, breast, and colorectal cancers. Black women had the highest breast cancer mortality rate (31.4/100,000), and the second highest rate of cervical cancer (6.7/100,000) and colorectal cancer.

Since 1973, the number of African-American women of all ages who have died from breast cancer has risen 18 percent. American black women are less likely to develop breast cancer, but are more likely to die from it than white American women.[1]

According to one study, socioeconomic factors, together with cultural beliefs, may account for the fact that black women tend to show more advanced-stage breast cancer than white women (30 percent for black women, compared to 12 percent for white women).[2]

Black women are less likely to develop breast cancer, endometrial cancer, and hip fractures than white women, but when black women develop these diseases, they are more likely to die from them. Black women are also more likely to develop heart disease than white females. There are a number of possible explanations for these patterns: detection bias, lack of access to education, and lack of access to preventive care programs. Or, this pattern may be due to more serious concerns: Is breast cancer simply more deadly among black women? There are no answers to any of these concerns; neither are there any definitive methods to prevent breast cancer. All women, regardless of race, should use all the information that is available to them to avoid this deadly disease.

Prevention of Breast Cancer

My friend Shirley Day Williams died of breast cancer at age 61. When she was initially diagnosed, many well-meaning friends offered various explanations. One of the many suggestions was that she was angry with herself and that the anger was manifesting itself as breast cancer. No one really knows what triggers cells in the breast to become cancerous. Lifestyle factors such as alcohol consumption, high-fat diets, cigarette smoking, and other environmental factors have been mentioned as possible contributors to breast cancer, but more studies are needed. Breast cancer can strike anyone, even those who have followed all the recommendations. A woman has no choice other than to do what has been proven so far to reduce her risk of breast cancer.

How to decrease your risk of breast cancer: It is not fully understood why some women develop breast cancer. Early detection with breast self-exams, mammograms, and other diagnostic modalities makes early treatment possible, with the best hope for a cure. Other preventive steps include a low-fat diet, avoiding obesity, and hormone replacement therapy. Tamoxifen shows promise in helping decrease the risk among women at high risk for developing breast cancer.

Some other facts to take into consideration concern . . .

— *Smoking:* Women who smoke cigarettes quadruple their risk of breast cancer.[3]

— *Alcohol:* A study of 322,647 women who consumed two to five alcoholic beverages (wine, beer, and hard liquor) per day demonstrated a 41 percent increased risk of developing invasive breast cancer. Women who drank one alcoholic beverage per day were also found to be at increased risk.

— *Nutrition:* Women who eat a diet rich in fruits and vegetables and who exercise are less likely to develop breast cancer and other cancers.[4]

Asian women who consumed fish oil, rich in omega-3 fatty acids, instead of vegetable oils, experience lower breast cancer rates.

— *Exercise:* Women who exercise regularly are less likely to develop breast cancer.[5, 6]

Estrogen replacement therapy: There is a lot of controversy about estrogen replacement therapy. Many studies have demonstrated that there is an increase in breast cancer risk, while others have not. The Women's Health Initiative Trial, sponsored by the National Institutes of Health, is searching for such an answer, but the clinical data will not be available until 2005. Meanwhile, women like you and I have to make the best of what's available.

— **Does estrogen, or the combination of estrogen and progestins, increase the chance of breast cancer?**

As mentioned above, studies on hormone replacement therapy and breast cancer are not clearly defined. Some research has shown that there is an increased risk of breast cancer with estrogen replacement therapy, and the longer the use, the greater the risk—while other research has shown otherwise. Additional studies have shown an increase of between 30 to 40 percent in the incidence of breast cancer after using HRT for more than ten years. For now, the prevailing belief is that there is a slight increase in the risk of breast cancer when taking HRT more than five years. As a counterbalance, according to one study, HRT, with its beneficial effects on cardiovascular mortality, would result in a net total of 302 lives saved per year for each 100,000 women aged 65 to 75 years. As you can see, the actual risk of cancer due to HRT has not been precisely quantified.

It should be noted that breast cancers in women on HRT are less aggressive. According to a study at the University of Tampere, Finland, women diagnosed with breast cancer while on HRT were found to have a significantly higher percentage of smaller and less aggressive tumors.

The breast cancer gene test: Among the general population, 6 out of every 10,000 women carry the BRCA-1 and BRCA-2 genes.[7] (These genes are more common among Jewish women of Ashkenazi decent).[8] According to the University of Pennsylvania, women who carry these genes and possess a strong family history of breast or ovarian cancer are at an increased risk of about 10 percent. A woman with a family history of breast cancer has a 7 in 100 chance of inheriting a mutated form of the BCRA-1. Now that BCRA-1 testing is available to detect the gene that predisposes women to breast and ovarian cancer, it is being requested often.

Women should be cautious about this test. First of all, the results of the screening are far from absolute. A positive test means that a woman is at a relatively high risk of developing familial breast or ovarian cancer—some studies have suggested as much as 5 to 15 percent. For a better perspective, 75 percent of women who develop breast cancer have no prior high-risk factors for the disease.

A woman may develop a false sense of security if the test comes back negative. There are other ramifications of the test result: If a woman tests positive, could she be denied health insurance in the future? The test is also costly; it is not covered by public, private, or managed-care organizations at this time. It costs about $1,000 for the first family member and $250 to $300 for each additional member, after a mutation has been identified.

— *Is genetic testing for you?* Four weeks after her mastectomy and breast reconstructive surgery, my patient Gina came to see me with her daughter, Karen, a 34-year-old single woman with no children. They were accompanied by Gina's mother, also my patient, a very healthy 84-year-old woman with no history of cancer. Gina was the first female in her family to have cancer. The women had heard about the breast and ovarian cancer gene tests. Their concern was that Karen was possibly at risk of developing ovarian and breast cancer because Gina had it. They were wondering if they should all take the gene tests to find out if they were carriers.

I asked Karen what she would do if the test results indicated that she was a carrier. Would she have a mastectomy or have her ovaries removed? Karen answered that her future plans included marriage and a family, regardless of the test results. She decided not to intervene at this time. In Karen's case, there was no reason to take the test now; she would wait until the necessity for testing became a higher priority.

Tamoxifen and breast cancer: Tamoxifen, like estrogen, locks onto estrogen receptors in the breast tissue, blocking or displacing estrogen, but without stimulating malignant cells. A large-scale, four-year American study, the Breast Cancer Prevention Trial, involving 13,388 women, from April 1992 to March 1998, found that women at high risk for breast cancer reduced their chance by 45 percent of getting the disease by taking Tamoxifen.

But soon afterwards, two studies published in the *Lancet,* a British medical journal, negated those findings. The first one, a smaller but longer-run study of eight years at the Royal Marsden Hospital in London, found the incidence of breast cancer among 2,494 women with a family history of the disease was the same regardless of whether they took the drug. The second study by the European Institute of Oncology in Milan, Italy, followed 5,408 women for four years and came to a similar conclusion.

Side effects of Tamoxifen include an increased risk of uterine cancer and blood clots. Women over the age of 50 are three times as likely to suffer blood clots in the legs; two women have died of such clots. These women also had twice the risk of cancer of the uterine lining and were treated with a hysterectomy. According to one researcher, "The frequency of the risk is much less than the frequency of the benefits."

The women in the Breast Cancer Prevention Trial were followed for only four years. The question remains: How long will the protective effects last, and for how long should the drug be taken? No one knows how to predict which women are at increased risk of developing deadly complications. Women are also supposed to take Tamoxifen for only five years. It is not known how long the benefits last once they stop therapy.

Women at a high risk for breast cancer need to make an informed decision. The National Women's Health Network states that it is premature to celebrate Tamoxifen as a prevention to breast cancer. More studies are needed.

Prophylactic mastectomy and breast cancer prevention: The removal of all breast tissue before cancer has a chance to develop is another option. According to a Mayo Clinic study, preventive bilateral mastectomy decreased the risk of developing breast cancer by up to 97 percent. However, there is still a small chance, estimated to be between 3 to 15 percent, of developing breast cancer after such a radical procedure.[9] Only a minority of high-risk women have undergone this procedure. Most of those who did went on to have their breasts reconstructed with implants.

Prophylactic mastectomy should be reserved for women who are at an extremely high risk for developing breast cancer, such as women who have had breast cancer in one breast, those with certain precancerous conditions of the breast, and those with a strong family history of breast cancer. Just like any other procedure, the decision to have a prophylactic mastectomy should be undertaken only after careful consideration by a woman and her health-care provider.

What Can a Woman Do to Detect Breast Cancer Early?

The breast exam: You should perform a breast self-exam regularly and note any changes in the breast—a lump, skin changes, or abnormal nipple discharge. If you note a change, make an appointment with your health-care provider as soon as possible. If you have a teenage daughter, be sure she learns how to do a breast self-exam.

— *Why perform a breast self-examination?* I have heard many excuses for why some women do not do a monthly breast self-exam. Some have confessed to me that they refuse to examine their breasts because they're afraid to find something wrong. Some said that they leave their breast exam to their partner. Some forget; some are too self-conscious.

The structure and position of the breasts changes throughout a woman's life. Puberty, pregnancy, hormones, menopause, and weight gain or loss can all cause breast changes. I went through a period myself, which I call my midlife crisis, when I stopped exercising and ate everything in sight. I slowly gained an excess of 25 pounds. My breasts also got bigger, and I was soon plagued with upper-back pain. With a more appropriate diet and exercise regimen, I eventually lost the weight. It took me six months. During this time, I noticed how my breasts had changed. By the time I lost the weight, my breasts were totally different. I had to reprogram in my mind where the new lumps and bumps were.

— ***When to do the breast exam***: Examining your breasts once each month is one of the most important steps in taking charge of your own health. The best time is a week after the start of your menstrual period. If you don't menstruate, choose an easy-to-remember date, such as the first of the month.

The self-exam consists of two distinct parts: inspection and palpation.

— ***How to do the breast inspection:*** In front of a mirror, first with your arms relaxed at your side, then with your hands on your hips, and then with your arms held straight above your head, note any changes as you move to different positions.

If your breasts are large and pendulous and raising your arms does not allow you to see their undersides, do the exercise this way: Stand with your side to a mirror and bend forward from the waist. Place your hands on your hips and check the bottom contour of your breast in the mirror for puckering, indentations, or any other changes. Now turn your other side to the mirror, and with your hands on your hips, check your other breast.

While showing one of my patients how to do her breast self-exam, she saw how difficult it was to see the undersides of her breasts. She commented, "Doc, I guess I have to stand on my head; otherwise, I don't see how you're going to make these breasts move." Every time she returns for her yearly checkup, we laugh all over again.

— ***How to do breast palpation:*** You will be looking for any changes from previous exams and any new lumps or thickening. In the shower, raise one arm and use the fingers of the opposite hand to feel the breast for any masses or unusual thickness. Do this for each breast.

After you're out of the shower, lie down on your back with a folded towel below one shoulder. Put one hand under your head, and feel the breast with the three middle fingers of the opposite hand. Using a circular and continuous motion, with varying pressure to sense the consistency of breast tissue at different depths under the skin, palpate the whole breast, beginning around the nipple. Without lifting the fingers, enlarge the circle until you have examined the entire breast. Then gently squeeze each nipple for any discharge or bleeding. Now perform the same sequence on the other breast.

When your health-care provider performs your annual exam, take the opportunity to demonstrate your self-exam technique to be sure you're doing it correctly.

Your annual breast exam: Another way to increase your chances of early breast cancer detection is to have a yearly breast exam done by your health-care provider. An annual examination has been shown to detect 10 percent of all breast cancers.[10] However, going to a health-care provider does not necessarily mean that you'll automatically receive a proper breast exam. Not all of them are comfortable performing breast examinations.

Most breast cancers are discovered by the patient herself. Since you are the one who is most familiar with your breasts, you will be more apt to appreciate any minor variation. If you feel that something is wrong and your health-care provider cannot feel or detect anything by mammogram or ultrasound, you should seek another opinion.

The Mammogram

The first time I faced having a mammogram, I dreaded it. After the mammogram, when a friend asked me to describe my experience, I did so with some difficulty. I took both of my hands and put them by my left breast while making a squeezing motion, first up and down, then side-to-side. It was like taking two books that have been in the freezer for a few hours, and squeezing your breasts with them. Fortunately, the Breast Care Center, where I refer most of my patients in San Diego, has a very warm and welcoming atmosphere, and the technologists and radiologists are very competent.

Like the pelvic exam, the mammogram is something we women have to endure. Some, like me, resent the fact that women have to deal with so much with respect to our bodies throughout their lives. I remind patients who voice this concern that men seem to have it easy while they are young, but their turn will soon come! They will spend the rest of their years consulting with the urologist about their prostate—and most men hate the rectal exam. Knowing this makes dealing with PMS, cramps, pelvic exams, and mammograms just a little easier!

On a serious note, during the mammogram, a special machine similar to an x-ray machine is positioned in front of each breast. Separately, each breast is placed on a plastic plate and briefly compressed. This compression is necessary in order to obtain a clear picture of the breast with the least amount of radiation. Two views are obtained for each breast, one from above and one from the side. In some instances, some additional views may be required. Like other x-rays, the films are studied by a radiologist who will share the results with your health-care provider within one to two days. It is usually recommended that no deodorant be used the day of the mammogram since it might contain particles that could interfere with the interpretation of the films. The entire procedure takes about half an hour.

If any abnormality is detected on the initial mammogram, you may be called in to have an additional test, such as a coned compression view or an ultrasound. During the coned compression view, the particular suspicious area is magnified for better visualization. Talk about contortions and compressions undergone during a regular mammogram—the coned compression is even worse! An ultrasound may sometimes be required to differentiate between a solid or cystic mass.

Over 50 percent of women who have had a mammogram complain of some type of discomfort due to the compression of the breast by the mammography machine. If the discomfort persists, take a mild analgesic such as Tylenol. Sometimes the skin is slightly discolored following a mammogram, but this usually disappears within a few days.

Kinds of mammograms: A screening mammogram is used to detect unsuspected breast cancer at an early stage in women with no symptoms. Diagnostic mammograms are used to evaluate symptomatic women. Diagnostic mammograms may require more views and other methods, such as an ultrasound for definitive diagnosis.

When is the best time to have a mammogram? If you are still menstruating, you should schedule your mammogram during the second week of your menstrual cycle. The breast of a woman in her 40s is also less dense during the follicular cycle, making the interpretation of a mammogram easier. Because of the hormonal changes that occur in the breasts before menstruation, they may be tender, and you may experience much unnecessary pain due to the squeezing that occurs if the procedure is performed at this time.

How often should you have a mammogram? It used to be that a woman would have a baseline mammogram at age 35, then every one or two years between the ages of 40 and 50, depending upon the woman's risk factors. This issue has been controversial for many years, and the evidence about the benefits of mammography has been contradictory for the past decade. Should mammograms be performed between the ages of 40 and 50? Some studies have shown that 25 percent of cancers discovered by mammograms are among women in this age group. In 1993, the National Cancer Institute held an international workshop that resulted in a policy statement not recommending mammographic screening for women under age 50. They concluded that among women aged 40 to 49, randomized controlled trials showed no benefits for screening for the first five to seven years. As of May 1997, the National Cancer Institute recommends that a mammogram be done every one to two years in women aged 40 to 49. The National Institutes of Health now has no single recommendation for mammography for all women in their 40s.

The American College of Obstetricians and Gynecologists recommends that a woman should have an initial, or baseline, mammogram beginning at the age of 40, then every other year until age 50. After age 50, a mammogram should be taken every year. Women aged 35 and older with a family history of premenopausally diagnosed breast cancer in a first-degree relative should have annual mammograms.

The American Cancer Society recommends that women in their 40s should have annual mammograms.

The overall consensus at present is to leave the decision to the woman and her health-care provider. Personally, I have a mammogram every other year; I am now in my late 40s. I have reviewed the literature at length and have some doubts myself. As Dr. Christiane Northrup says, "A woman has to trust her inner wisdom." Having a mammogram every other year seems to be the right choice for me. I advise my patients who are in their 40s to do what feels right for them. Some have chosen to have one every other year, some once a year. *Basically, each woman has to decide for herself whether to undergo mammography.*

Limitations of mammography: Mammograms have been promoted as the solution to early detection of breast cancer, but they are not. Since the 1930s, there has been little change in the death rate from breast cancer, despite the advances in mammography technology and treatments such as chemotherapy. By the time a tumor is detected by a mammogram, it has often been growing for at least five years. More research is needed to find better methods for early breast cancer detection.

False-positive mammograms: One in ten women will be asked to return for further procedures such as the coned compression view or ultrasound. According to a study, if a woman has a yearly mammogram between the ages of 40 and 50, there is a 50-50 chance that she will have a false-positive mammogram. False positives increase the rate of biopsies. About 10 percent of mammograms require further evaluation. This can be very frightening. It happened to me once. When I got the phone call, I panicked. I was not the doctor who knew that it would probably be benign, and if there was something wrong, I would have a better chance since it would have been caught early. No, I was a scared patient just like anyone else. Fortunately, everything checked out okay.

A Patient's Story

Recently I had a 48-year-old patient, Sally, who had to return for further x-rays because some suspicious calcifications were noted on her mammogram. (Sally had no history of breast cancer in her family.) Typically, I will receive the mammogram report by mail. So, when I received a call from Louise O'Shaugnessy, the radiologist who usually reads my personal mammograms, I knew something was wrong. This call had to do with Sally's mammogram results. In her case, a stereotactic biopsy was indicated and could be performed the next morning, with the result promised the following day.

That night, I called Sally at home and comforted her. She was very anxious about her upcoming procedure; obviously she was very worried that we would find something wrong with her. The day after the surgery, as promised, I got a call from Dr. Tony Iagmin, the pathologist; it was benign calcification. I was so relieved. I called Sally at work and told her that the biopsy was benign. She said, "You know, you saved my sanity and my life." As I hung up the phone, I said, "I know."

False-negative mammograms: In women with dense breasts, such as younger women and those on hormone replacement therapy, there is a low proportion of fatty tissue. Among these women, there is a 10 to 15 percent incidence of false-negative results, meaning that the mammogram appears normal even though cancer is present. As many as 10 to 30 percent of palpable cancers do not show up on mammograms. This is more likely to occur in women under age 50. When a new lump is found during a breast self-exam or by a health-care provider, it should be biopsied, even though the mammogram comes up negative.

A PATIENT'S STORY

Alice, a 62-year-old patient of mine, usually had her mammogram done before her exam, except for this time. During the breast inspection, I noticed a small puckering the size of a pencil eraser about three inches below her left nipple. While I was palpating this area, my fingers perceived a slight thickening, but no definite mass. I guided Alice's hand to the site and asked her if she noticed any changes. She did not. I had a strange feeling that something was wrong. I took a mirror and asked her if she could see what I was pointing to, but she could not.

I told Alice that I wanted her to have a mammogram right away. On the request form, I drew a picture of a breast and put an X on the area of concern. I wrote: "Very suspicious for malignancy." I also recommended that she see a surgeon and have the area biopsied, regardless of the mammographic findings.

Alice went for her mammogram, and the first routine films were normal. The technician could not palpate any mass but had to go by my request form. She then called the radiologist, who could not find anything either. They did a "coned down" or magnified views of the area that I had marked, and only then noticed the area that looked "somewhat suspicious."

When Alice went to see the surgeon, he could neither palpate nor see anything. I received a note from the surgeon telling me he was going to do an excisional biopsy of the area, using the fine-needle localization method.

I was shocked when I received the pathological report of the breast biopsy and mastectomy. Alice had a one and one-half centimeter cancer, and all of the nodes were negative. I called Alice at home to find out what was going on. Before the excisional biopsy, Alice was given the choice between a lumpectomy and a mastectomy, if it turned out to be cancer. She chose a mastectomy, because in her mind, there was nothing wrong. She was so sure that she would wake up with just a little scar on her breast from the biopsy.

When she got home two days later, Alice noted that the left side of her chest, including the scar, was turning black and blue. She had been taking Daypro, an aspirin-like medication that was apparently mistaken for a vitamin. Alice had to be readmitted for drainage of a large hematoma and required two units of blood.

When I saw Alice a few weeks later for something else, I noticed that her breast area still looked bad. Mentally, Alice felt okay about her decision. "I am without a breast, but it's okay, and my husband is very supportive. At least I don't have to go through radiation therapy."

Alice came back a few months later. She was now very self-conscious about her missing breast, but she did not want to go through a breast reconstruction procedure. I referred her to Bink, a certified mastectomy fitter. A breast cancer survivor herself, Bink is the owner of a store in San Diego called "The Brighter Side." In her boutique, women with cancer can find nonmedical products that are needed during and after treatment.

Alice called me after her visit to the boutique. She was very happy, as she had bought a permanent silicone breast form that she puts in her bra to give her a natural, weighted feeling.

It has been five years, and Alice is cancer-free. She opted not to take Tamoxifen. I always wondered what would have happened if she was someone else's patient at the time of the false-negative mammogram.

What about radiation risk with mammograms? The radiation dose of a mammogram equals the radiation exposure received from two round-trip flights between the East and West Coasts of the United States. Only one out of a million women may develop breast cancer because of mammogram procedure radiation.[11]

Mammograms and breast implants: Women who have breast implants are usually concerned about their implants rupturing during a mammogram. I have always reassured them that this is a rare occurrence, until it happened to a patient of mine named Booie.

A PATIENT'S STORY

Booie was very flat-chested before having saline implants. Three days after she'd had her mammogram, she noticed her right breast getting smaller and smaller, until finally it flattened out. She was emotionally distraught and concerned that whatever was in the implant was being absorbed throughout her body. Her husband, trying to be a good sport, jokingly told her not to worry—she just had a flat tire and could go back to the doctor and have it pumped up again. Booie found out that she could not just have saline reinjected into the breast; she had to have the old implant removed and replaced with a new one. She was undecided. Should she just have both implants removed? When she considered the extreme difference in size and attractiveness, as well as the idea of having to go through two different procedures, she opted to have the implant replaced.

(According to a long-term follow-up study of more than 3,000 women with breast implants, it has been documented that breast implants do not raise the risk of cancer.)

Micro-calcification on mammograms: Micro-calcification, tiny specks of calcium that appear on a mammogram, are common. Eighty percent of micro-calcifications are not a precursor to cancer. When discovered in a first mammogram, they will have to be followed by another mammogram in six months. If a micro-calcification looks suspicious, it should be biopsied. My patient Gina's breast cancer was discovered when her screening mammogram showed some abnormal calcifications.

Please remember:

- If you have a personal history of breast cancer, or if you have had an abnormal breast biopsy result, you need to have a mammogram every year after diagnosis or your biopsy.

- If your mother, sister, or daughter had breast cancer before age 50, you need to have a mammogram every year starting at age 35.

- If your mother, sister, or daughter had breast cancer at age 50 or older, you need to have a mammogram every year starting at age 40.

- Most breast lumps are benign; only two out of ten breast lumps turn out to be cancerous.

- Recovery from breast cancer is very high if detected early.

- A bloody discharge from the nipple may be associated with cancer.

- Trauma to the breast does not cause breast cancer.

- Examine your breasts every month. Inspection of your breasts in front of a mirror is an important part of your breast self-exam. Make sure to note any changes in the skin, contour of the breast, and any nipple changes.

- Have a complete physical exam every year, including a breast exam.

- Try to have each mammogram at the same facility so that subtle changes can be detected.

- Mammograms can miss 10 to 15 percent of all breast cancers. If you find a new lump, it should be biopsied regardless of the mammogram result.

- Alert others to cancer information and the importance of breast examinations.

- Take charge of your body. Your health is in your hands.

- Overall, there is no doubt that prevention is the best medicine. If cancer does strike, know that you are not alone. You can get help. Do not be afraid to ask.

- Be sure that whomever performs your mammogram is certified to do so!

- Keep informed about cancer research treatment. (Please check my website at **www.drcarolle.com** for updated information and research results.)

BREAST HEALTH MADE EASY
(A quick summary on how to maintain breast health)

- Examine your breasts on a monthly basis—
  report any abnormal findings to your health-care provider
- Have a yearly breast exam done by your health-care provider
- Get a mammogram regularly (40 to 50 years old—have a mammogram every one to two years; 50 years and older—have a mammogram every year)
- Start an exercise program
- Stop smoking
- Use alcohol in moderation
- Keep your weight under control
- Eat healthfully and take nutritional supplements

CHAPTER 9

Alzheimer's Disease

A lzheimer's is the most common of disorders causing cognitive decline in old age, and it accounts for about 50 percent of all cases of dementia. In its early stages, Alzheimer's can be confused with depression—patients experience withdrawal, loss of concentration, memory failures, delusion, agitation, intellectual impairment, and anxiety. As the disease progresses, an individual may become extremely confused, unaware of her surroundings, disoriented, suspicious, paranoid, fearful, irritable, and even violent. During the latter stages, people may become unable to take care of themselves and may be unable to socialize or communicate. The impact of an elderly parent with Alzheimer's is greater for women because they are usually the caretakers.

Most Alzheimer's occurs later in life, with a greater prevalence after age 65. Approximately 10 percent of Americans older than 65 have the disease; almost 50 percent of those sufferers are over the age of 85. Alzheimer's occurs more often among women than men, partially because women typically outlive men.

The cause of Alzheimer's disease is unknown. Multiple factors including environmental influences, nutritional deficiencies, and genetic factors may contribute to the disease. In 1993, a specific protein was isolated as a factor.

Some possible causes of Alzheimer's disease have been postulated to be:

- hypertension
- diabetes
- alcoholism
- a history of hypothyroidism, head trauma, hip fractures, myocardial infarction, or strokes
- having had general anesthesia
- estrogen deficiency
- carrying an apolipoprotein E4 allele

Studies have also revealed that higher levels of education and intelligence are related to a decreased risk of Alzheimer's disease.

Diagnosis of Alzheimer's Disease

This disease is difficult to diagnose, especially during the early stages, and it can often be misdiagnosed. According to some experts, the only real way to diagnose Alzheimer's is with a brain biopsy—which is performed after death. The diagnosis may be based upon symptoms described by family members or the individual. Some tests are available, though, that can evaluate an individual's level of mental functioning. Occasionally, a magnetic resonance imaging (MRI) or a computed tomography (CT) scan of the brain may reveal some changes that are associated with the disease.

Alzheimer's Disease's Prevention

- If you smoke, here is another reason you should quit: Cigarette smoking causes small blood vessel damage that decreases oxygen to the brain.

- Regular exercise has been shown to improve memory in women with dementia.

- Stay active, be involved with life, and be a constant learner.

- Antioxidants reduce the amount of free-radicals in brain tissue and may have a beneficial effect against Alzheimer's disease.[1]

- Other strategies include the use of nonsteroidal anti-inflammatory medications such as ibuprofen.

- Women who take estrogen can slow age-related memory loss and possibly prevent Alzheimer's disease.

Treatment of Alzheimer's Disease

There is no cure for Alzheimer's disease. The drug Tacrine can slow the progression of the disease, but not by very much. It also has some severe side effects, such as nausea, vomiting, and liver damage. Another drug, Aricept, can help reduce memory loss but eventually loses effectiveness. Vitamin E, 200 IU per day, may delay functional deterioration among patients with Alzheimer's. High doses of vitamin E, as much as 2,000 IU, may also delay the progression of dementia.

A study published in *JAMA* demonstrated that the herb ginkgo biloba may help delay the progression of dementia among some elderly patients. This benefit lasted from six months to a year.

Estrogen has been found to have multiple actions in the brain that may have an important effect on Alzheimer's disease.[2] Estrogen also enhances or maintains mood and memory.[3] Other studies suggest that long-term estrogen may decrease the incidence or severity of Alzheimer's disease.[4] More studies are needed. (Please check my website at **www.drcarolle.com** for updated information and research results.)

PART II

Lifestyle Changes

As we noted in Part I, there are a number of factors that affect and involve menopause. The choice a woman makes for her particular situation will be dependent on those factors, as well as risk factors due to age, family history, genetics, culture, and race. For many women, conventional medicine doesn't have all the answers. Many studies have shown that modifying one's lifestyle, including proper nutrition, supplements, regular exercise, stress reduction, relaxation, prevention of sexually transmitted diseases, smoking cessation, alcohol and drug use, maintaining a normal body weight, and regular checkups can reduce many of these risk factors, which we'll discuss in this section and also cover in Part III, "For Further Reference."

CHAPTER 10

Stress and Depression

Stress is something that Mother Nature built into us way back in evolutionary times to prepare us to meet and survive the unexpected. Stress induces the "fight or flight" response, enabling us to overpower our enemies or escape from them. When we react to something we perceive as dangerous, the body pumps out hormones that make us more alert and ready to act. The heart beats faster, blood pressure increases, and muscles tense. If we act on these signals with our physical body—by running or fighting—the excess energy is used up.

In our modern society, stress can impact us at work or at home, although not usually in the form of a lurking saber-toothed tiger! Stress keeps pumping hormones into the bloodstream until they assault the blood vessels, the heart, the immune system, and the liver. This can produce problems such as high blood pressure, increased susceptibility to illness,[1] viral and bacterial infections,[2] ulcers, headaches, chronic muscular tension, high cholesterol levels, heart attacks, hormonal imbalance,[3] and even cancer.[4] Among women, it can also cause menstrual irregularities.

Unsuspected Stress

Many life events, both the positive and the negative, can precipitate stress. Some examples of stressful triggers are getting married or divorced;

bearing children; children moving away from home; changes in partners; a chronic illness (or a partner with one); shifts in financial status; changing or losing a job; the death of a friend or family member; moving, selling, or buying a home; accidents; and environmental stressors; to name but a few.

A Personal Story

Another stressor that few people recognize until it happens is the loss of an animal companion. I never had a pet growing up, and didn't realize just how attached a person could become to a dog until my ex-husband, Thomas, acquired Czar, a most beautiful and intelligent German shepherd. Czar became my best friend. This was the first time I experienced what is often referred to as unconditional love. When I had to put him to sleep after seven years because he had cancer of the spine, it was the most painful thing that I've ever had to do. I cried and cried for a long time. This was a new stressful event in my life.

Some patients have come into my office with many symptoms suggestive of stress. After talking with them for a while, I would sometimes discover that they had recently lost an animal companion. Talking about the loss helped them to realize that they had been more affected than they realized.

Women and Stress

Women naturally need close relationships such as family members, friends, or a partner in order to thrive. It has been documented that a woman's ability to nurture relationships, which includes social support from others, can benefit her both physically and mentally.

Women are more vulnerable to stress than men. We have been raised to become caretakers, good mothers, and spouses, and to care for our elderly parents and animal companions. When we begin to feel overwhelmed and ask for help, we are often told that we're being selfish. People around us know very well how to play with our guilt. Black women more than white women are expected to be strong and to take care of the "whole race." Also, black women are less likely to seek counseling.

There are two types of stress, negative and positive. The difference between the two depends upon whether you feel you are in *control* of the stress. Some stress helps you focus your energies, sort out your priorities, make decisions, and perform better—this is positive stress. Negative stress occurs when you feel a lack of control over a particular situation.

Negative stress is what invariably happens to women. Women are less prone to be in positions of power to control what happens in their lives. Women also tend to take care of everyone else's needs before taking care of their own. I have many patients who are symptomatic with advanced cancer. When I ask why they had not come in sooner, the typical answer is that they were busy caring for an elderly parent, a sick spouse, or their children.

Women are also expected to perform multiple tasks and duties. They often hold a full-time job, and then come home and cook dinner and take care of the household. Women sometimes place themselves in this position; they maintain relationships with partners, relatives, and children who all have needs and expectations. Women may speak up and complain that the husband or the teenager does not help. Why should they? They know that she will complain, and then she will do the task herself! When I ask women why they continue to do so, they don't know the answer. They feel like they have to, unaware that they are becoming stressed and resentful.

Warning Signs of Stress

Physical signs: Stress can affect you physically, emotionally, and behaviorally. Listen to your body to recognize some of these physical signs of stress.

- Excessive heartburn
- Lack of appetite, or overeating
- Gastritis
- Stomach or duodenal ulcers
- Ulcerative colitis
- Irritable bowel
- Absence of menses (if you are not menopausal)
- Irregular menses
- Loss of hair (alopecia areata)
- Mouth ulcers
- Trouble falling asleep
- Nightmares
- Irregular heartbeat after a period of stress
- Anxiety attack
- Tension headaches
- Muscle spasms
- Trembling or shaking
- Inability to concentrate
- Chronic fatigue
- Skin disorders
- Teeth grinding

Women frequently come to my office complaining of lower abdominal pain severe enough for me to perform a diagnostic laparoscopy to look for pelvic inflammatory disease, or endometriosis (when the lining of the uterus is present in other parts of the pelvis, causing scarring and pain)—only to find a perfectly normal pelvis. Some women who are under stress will suffer bouts of constipation or diarrhea and bloating. Others may experience some of the symptoms mentioned above. High levels of consistent stress can also cause hypertension.

When a woman who has been having irregular periods comes to see me, many times I find out that the culprit is stress. This even happened to me. During my third year of residency training, I spent two months during the winter of 1980 at the University of Madison, Wisconsin (UMW). The chief of the Department of Reproductive Endocrinology was blatantly racist, sexist, and had an aversion to foreign medical students. While working under this man, my period disappeared and did not return for two months.

When I am under stress, I tend to have severe lower abdominal cramping and bloating, as well as a sharp pain in my lower right side. This started while I was in medical school. The first time it happened, I was preparing for finals. One night I awoke with pain so severe that I thought that I must have appendicitis. I was rushed to the emergency room, poked, and told that all the tests were negative. When it happened again, during my residency training, it was so severe that I went to see my gynecologist. He knew I must be in bad shape; two months prior, during my routine exam, I had told him how I hated coming to see him!

High levels of stress can increase your susceptibility to illness. Chronic emotional stress results in the suppression of the immune system, which in turn, increases the susceptibility to immune-related disorders. Stress can also aggravate conditions such as arthritis, asthma, emphysema, neuromuscular syndromes, atherosclerosis, and skin disorders.

Behavioral signs: While under stress, some women tend to develop eating disorders such as anorexia, overeating, or bulimia. They also have a tendency to abuse illicit and prescription drugs, alcohol, and cigarettes. Some women who've quit smoking may resume the habit at this time. Women who are under a lot of stress are more likely to experience stress-related illnesses and may be more prone to accidental injuries. They may perform poorly at work and tend to be involved in more interpersonal problems, family conflicts, and social isolation. Women who are stressed are also more likely to suffer from the common cold.

Emotional signs: Some women experience difficulty concentrating while under stress. During my so-called midlife crisis, one of the first symptoms I experienced was forgetfulness. I missed freeway exits and let the water run in the backyard until a neighbor called. Other signs include anxiety, irritability, difficulty falling asleep, and staying asleep.

Controlling Stress

You can't totally eliminate stress from your life, so the secret is learning how to *control* it, working with it to your advantage. People who don't know how to control stress in a positive manner typically revert to unhealthy alternatives—drinking, smoking, drug abuse, overeating, promiscuity, or overwork. Stress can also cause people to mentally or physically abuse their children or spouse. It has even been linked to motor-vehicle accidents.

Dealing with stress is difficult for women and can be even harder for men. It's okay for a woman to cry, to admit something is wrong, to seek solace from a friend, or to enlist professional help. Prevailing American attitudes make it very difficult for men to ask for help.

Fortunately, there are many ways to relieve stress:

- If you're constantly tired or fatigued, you may be suffering from an underactive thyroid. A simple, inexpensive blood test that will detect a malfunctioning thyroid can be ordered by your doctor.

- Think about what stresses you, and make a list. A few years ago, I went through what I called my midlife crisis. I saw a therapist, Denise, who asked me to list everything that I felt was stressing me. She had me keep a journal in which I wrote what came to mind about stressful situations that could not be changed at the time.

- Learn your warning signs of stress. When they appear, take a break. I realized that my lower abdominal cramping and bloating occurred when I was under a lot of stress.

- Exercise regularly. I have an exercise routine that I maintain. After a workout, I find that little things that used to bother me are irrelevant.

- Try some relaxation techniques such as meditation,[5] progressive muscle relaxation, stretching, guided visual imagery, biofeedback,[6] yoga,[7] and prayer. Also, you might find a nice bubble bath or a soak in a relaxing spa a simple stress reducer.

- Listen to relaxing music. When I drive, I don't listen to the news; I play music that I like on the radio or play instrumental or New Age tapes or CDs.

- Get a massage. If you can't afford it, ask your friends, co-workers, children, or partner to buy you one for your next birthday or holiday, instead of buying you a gift that you do not need.

- Join a self-help support group. Self-help groups offer a place to meet regularly and share experiences, and help you feel less alone.

- Get an adequate amount of sleep each night.

- Follow a sound nutritional program.

- Discontinue bad habits such as smoking. Avoid stimulants such as caffeine, herbs that contain ma huang and Chinese ephedra, and illegal drugs such as amphetamines and cocaine. Do not abuse alcohol.

- Herbs such as chamomile tea, passion flower, valerian root, and American ginseng are very good for relaxation.

- Stop watching the news on TV. Read the newspaper headlines and only those articles that interest you. Lately, I have not watched TV except to check the weather forecast!

- Maintain a clean and peaceful environment, and play soothing music at home.

- Breathe. When we're stressed, we tend to take quick, shallow breaths. To reduce stress, take slow, deep breaths; inhale deeply filling the entire diaphragm, and hold for a few seconds, then release the air very gradually. The result can be excellent for your mind and body.

- Talk to your good friends; recovery through my midlife crisis would have taken longer if I did not have good friends to talk to.

- Avoid going into debt. Don't buy what you cannot pay for.

- Try to keep a sense of humor.

- Take up a new hobby, join a club, or get an animal companion.

- Learn to set priorities, and only do what is most important. Find the time to do something for yourself—without feeling guilty. Some women find it difficult to relax, especially if they have a busy lifestyle and small children. Women are often caregivers to husbands, children, parents, and relatives. Who is last in line for receiving attention and nurturing? Women. I suggest that my patients try to see themselves as a battery that needs to be recharged from time to time. If it doesn't get recharged, the battery (like the woman) runs out of power just when it's needed most.

- Limit what must be done every day; there is always tomorrow.

- Start delegating responsibilities. Expect your children, especially teenagers, to do more things, and, in the process, teach them about responsibility.

- Learn how to say no to another task. Stop feeling guilty when you tell others that you cannot do what they ask.

A PERSONAL STORY

One day, Cynthia, a patient of mine for many years, came in for her annual exam. Just like me, she was going through what we called our midlife crisis, and she was learning how to cope. Suddenly, I had a brilliant idea. What about doing something spontaneous that I had never done for myself? What about just taking off and doing nothing!

"What are you going to do tomorrow?" I asked Cynthia. "Nothing," she said. So, I asked her to join me in a beautiful area of San Diego called Seaport Village just to goof off. She could not believe her ears.

When Cynthia and I met the next day, it was two o'clock in the afternoon. She told me she had been calling all her friends, telling them that she had an appointment by the ocean with her doctor to learn how to relax.

She was pulling into the parking lot at the same time I was arriving. We parked next to each other and headed to a Greek restaurant. We ate while giggling, like two young kids. We had our parking ticket validated for two hours of free parking. Each of us had brought a comfortable blanket, so we headed to a nice area on the grass by the ocean and plopped down, using our purses as pillows. It was a gorgeous day like so many are in San Diego. We spent the time watching the seagulls, yachts, and tourists, trying to find objects in the few clouds in the sky, and shooing away the peddlers who wanted to sell us something. How could we be depressed?

Depression

Depression is defined as a feeling of sadness, reduced activity, apathy, and self-deprecation. It is normal to feel sad from time to time; however, if the feeling persists for a long period of time and it's extreme, it could indicate a major physical or emotional problem that may require therapeutic intervention.

In the United States, the lifetime risk of major depression disorder among women ranges from 10 to 25 percent, compared with 2 to 3 percent for men. Each year, 20 million American adults experience a major depressive episode. Thirty-five percent of women, or one in three, experience a major depressive episode at some time over the course of their lifetime. Seventy percent of women experience mild to moderate mood and behavioral changes with their menstrual cycle; for 5 percent of these women, the symptoms can be so severe as to interfere with the quality of their life.

Perimenopause and menopause can be a time of increased depressive symptomatology, due to the presence of vasomotor symptoms such as hot flashes and night sweats, which cause disturbed sleep. If these symptoms persist over a period of time, they may cause chronic fatigue, which in turn can cause feelings of depression.

Magazine advertisements for Prozac encourage us to believe that if we are sad or irritable, have difficulty concentrating, have lost our appetite, lack energy, or have trouble feeling pleasure, we may be depressed and should seek treatment. I ask myself how many times I've felt these things. Many times. Was I depressed and in need of medication? No! Yet, antidepressants such as Prozac, Zoloft, and Paxil are selling like hotcakes.

(My editor told me that she went to her health maintenance organization [HMO] to get something for her PMS-related mood swings, and the doctor suggested Prozac. She angrily exclaimed that she didn't want to take something *every* day for something she only experienced a few days a month—and not every month at that! She ended up taking vitamins on her own.)

Some patients now go to their health-care providers, having self-diagnosed themselves, and demand a specific drug. Some health-care providers, especially HMOs, may give in too easily. When I have a patient who is under stress, I do not just hand her a prescription. I take the time to find out what the cause of her stress is and teach her how to deal with it. This may take two or three visits; if more time is needed, I refer her to a therapist.

I have also observed that here in America, we are raising a generation of misguided teenagers, especially among the white, middle-class population. They believe that life is supposed to be rosy, and if it isn't, it can be corrected with a pill. I cringe when I hear a teenager tell me she's taking antidepressants because she's "depressed." Instead of learning coping skills, these teenagers are popping pills. It is very sad.

I do admit that there are true cases of depression caused by a chemical imbalance that warrant prescription drugs, especially when the patient expresses suicidal thoughts. My feeling is that these cases are not as prevalent as the amount of drugs being prescribed would lead us to believe. Women should resist using antidepressants unless absolutely necessary, as determined by a comprehensive evaluation with a therapist or physician.

(According to one study, a major side effect of depression may be low bone density.[8] The pathophysiology is unknown. It seems that depressed women with low bone density may have a higher secretion of cortisol, a hormone secreted by the adrenal gland, closely related to cortisone in physiological effect.)

Mild depression: The symptoms of mild clinical depression include having a depressed mood for most of the day for at least two years, and experiencing at least two of the following symptoms:

- Sleeping problems: insomnia or oversleeping
- Changes in appetite: eating too much or not at all
- Changes in weight
- Fatigue or lack of energy
- Feelings of hopelessness, helplessness, and sadness
- Feeling guilty, worthless, or useless
- Difficulty concentrating, thinking, or making decisions

— *Treatment of mild depression:* The following treatments have been found to be helpful in the event of mild depression:

- Regular exercise
- Relaxation techniques such as meditation, progressive muscle relaxation, yoga, and biofeedback
- Mind/body interventions
- Dance and music

Following a healthy diet and taking vitamin B complex, folic acid, and selenium 100 mcg/day have also been found to be helpful. German studies have demonstrated that St. John's wort is as effective as Prozac for the treatment of mild depression, and it's less toxic. The recommended dosage is 300 mg, three times per day. **Caution:** Dosages over 900 mg per day may be harmful.

Severe Depression: The symptoms of severe clinical depression include a morose mood, a loss of interest in recreational activities, jobs, hobbies, friends, and sex, plus at least five of the following:

- Daily sleeping problems: too much or too little sleep
- Changes in appetite: eating too much or not eating at all
- Marked changes in weight

- Feeling blue and/or disinterested
- Difficulty concentrating, thinking, or making decisions
- Feelings of hopelessness, helplessness, or sadness
- Feelings of self-reproach or guilt
- Anxiety attacks
- Fatigue or loss of energy nearly every day
- Suicidal thoughts or recurring thoughts of death

— ***Treatment of severe depression:*** St John's wort may also be effective in the treatment of both moderate and severe depression.[9]

Both medication and psychotherapy have been found to be effective for the treatment of severe depression. Several types of antidepressants are available, which work by increasing the effectiveness of brain neurotransmitters. It typically requires six to eight weeks for antidepressant therapy to reveal its effectiveness.

Antidepressants are divided into several major groups:

- Tricyclics: Norpramin, Pamelor, Tofranil, Elavil, Vivactil, and Sinequan

- Selective Serotonin Reuptake Inhibitors (SSRIs): Prozac, Zoloft, Paxil, and Luvox

- Monoamine Oxidase Inhibitors (MAOIs): Marplan, Parnate, and Nardil

- Other classes (Wellbutrin and Desyrel).

Antidepressants should only be taken as prescribed, and you should be monitored closely by your health-care provider while you're taking them. Side effects vary with each drug, and are the most common reason for switching from one brand to another. If you are severely depressed, you should immediately seek medical attention.

CHAPTER 11

Implement a Healthy
Nutrition Program

What Is a Healthy Diet?

You probably already know that diet plays an important role in maintaining good health. What you eat and drink affects your risk of contracting heart disease, diabetes, cancer, stroke, and chronic liver disease. The immune system, which helps the body fight infection, requires the nutrients, minerals, and vitamins found in a healthy, balanced diet. But what is a healthy diet?

A healthy diet contains moderate amounts of protein (meat, fish, eggs, nuts, seeds, grain and bean combinations, and tofu). Proteins contain four calories per gram. Proteins are an essential part of the structure of every living cell and are responsible for physical development and growth.

A healthy diet is low in refined sugar and salt. The healthy diet is also rich in fiber. Fibers are substances that are not digestible in our diet, but provide bulk that helps our digestive system break down and assimilate food smoothly.

The healthy diet also contains carbohydrates, our best source of energy. There are two kinds of carbohydrates: complex carbohydrates such as cereals, wheat flour, rice, corn, pasta, beans, and vegetables; and simple carbohydrates, which are found in table sugar, white flour, honey, and fruits. Carbohydrates contain four calories per gram.

A healthy diet is low in fat. Fats contain nine calories per gram, more calories per unit than any other food. Fat isn't always bad for your health by any means, though. It helps provide the energy supply that the body needs in order to function. Women naturally have a higher percentage of fat in the body than men, and they need a certain amount to maintain a healthy level of estrogen, the main female hormone that controls the menstrual cycle.

The different types of fats that we consume in our diet are saturated fats, trans-fatty acids, monosaturated fats, polyunsaturated fat, and fish oils. It is not the *amount* of fat that you consume that is bad, but the *type* of fat. A high intake of saturated fat and trans-fatty acids increases the risk of cardiovascular disease, whereas monosaturated and polyunsaturated fat decrease the risk.[1]

Saturated fats: Saturated fats are primarily found in animal foods and tropical oils such as palm and coconut oils. Some studies have revealed a link between saturated fat and heart disease. There is also a link between saturated fat and a higher risk of breast cancer.[2] Some saturated fat is necessary for the liver's production of cholesterol.

Trans-fatty acids: Trans-fatty acids are found in margarine, commercially baked goods, and foods fried with hardened vegetable oil. Currently, 5 to 10 percent of fat in the American diet is trans-fatty acids. Trans-fatty acids are produced when vegetable oils are artificially hydrogenated to increase their firmness and resistance to rancidity. The softer the fat, the fewer trans-fatty acids it contains.

Monosaturated fats: Monosaturated fats, found in olive and canola oils, are considered healthier because of their ability to lower LDL, the "bad" cholesterol, while maintaining or raising HDL cholesterol. In places where olive oil is used as a fat, the populations have a lower incidence of heart disease and cancer.

Polyunsaturated fats: Polyunsaturated fats are found in safflower, sunflower, and corn oils, and they contain omega-6 and omega-3 essential fatty acids. In places where they are consumed, there is a decrease in the risk of heart disease and the incidence of arthritis, stroke, and some types of cancer.

Fish oils: Fish is rich in omega-3 fatty acids, eichosapentaenoic acid (EPA), and docosahexaenoic acid (DHA). These acids have beneficial effects on many body functions, which include reducing high lipids, blood pressure, and preventing blood clots.

People who eat a Mediterranean diet, which mainly consists of mono-saturated fat such as olive oil and canola oil, have a lower incidence of heart disease. This is true for the Eskimos and the Japanese, who consume large amounts of fish oil and fish in their diet.

One Australian study, published in *JAMA*, followed 9,014 males and females. Findings demonstrated that a moderate restriction of total and saturated dietary fat can be effective. No added benefits have been demonstrated with aggressive fat reduction, which could actually be counterproductive, since it may also lower HDL levels.

According to another study, a diet low in fat and higher in carbohydrates increases the risk of heart disease and stroke among postmenopausal women. Saturated fat should be replaced with monosaturated and polyunsaturated fats, rather than carbohydrates.[3]

Antioxidants and Health

Many studies have demonstrated that an adequate dietary intake of antioxidants may decrease your chances of developing heart disease, stroke, and various kinds of cancer. As your body uses the food you eat and the oxygen you breathe, a number of molecules (called "free radicals") are formed that damage healthy cells as they search for a component that will let them remain chemically independent. This process of oxidation—the attempt to attach missing electrons—wears down cell walls and alters the cell's DNA (basic genetic material). These changes can start the cell on the road to becoming cancerous.

Antioxidants are vitamins and minerals that neutralize free radicals by lending them electrons so they don't have a chance to damage the cells. Here are the corresponding food sources for some antioxidants. (See Table 11-b for recommended amounts.)

Vitamin A—liver, kidney, egg yolks, spinach, dairy products, cantaloupes, peaches, squash, all green and yellow fruits and vegetables

Beta carotene—raw carrots, cantaloupes, peaches, broccoli, cauli-flower, apricots, mangoes, squash, sweet potatoes, collard greens, kale, and carrots

Vitamin E—though hard to get from a standard diet, it can be found in most vegetables, wheat germ, safflower, sunflower, and soybeans oils; and in smaller amounts in peaches and prunes

Selenium—organ meats and seafood, garlic, grains, and mushrooms

Zinc—oysters, nettles, pumpkin seeds, spirulina, wild yams, legumes, and whole grains

Vitamin C—broccoli, cantaloupe, fresh tomatoes, oranges, orange juice, potatoes, raw green peppers, and strawberries

Allicin—garlic

Capsaicin—hot peppers

Lignans—flaxseed and wheat

Lycopene—tomatoes and red grapefruit

Drinking six to eight, eight-ounce glasses of liquid a day is also good for your health. Plain water is the best. Avoid caffeinated drinks such as cof-fee, tea, and cola beverages. Caffeine intake increases calcium excretion in the urine, which may lead to bone loss. Colas are also high in phosphorus, which adversely affects the bone. Beverages are also high in sugar—empty calories that you cannot afford!

Phytoestrogens

There is growing evidence that phytoestrogens, or plant estrogens, can provide important health benefits for women. Phytoestrogen is a naturally occurring plant sterol that has an effect similar to estrogen. Phytoestrogens are found in soybeans, flaxseed, legumes (dried peas and beans), red clover sprouts, and a number of fruits and vegetables. Asian women, especially the Japanese, experience a much lower incidence of hot flashes, heart disease, and osteoporotic fractures than American women because soy is a staple in their diet. The Japanese consume about 200 mg of soy per day, compared to the average Asian diet of 25 to 45 mg, and the average Western diet of 3 mg.

The beneficial effect of phytoestrogens comes from the isoflavones that are contained in soy products. Soy proteins contain the isoflavones diadzen and genestein, as well as essential amino acids, omega-3 fatty acids, calcium, and very little fat. Genestein in soy has been found to block tyrosine kinase, an enzyme needed for cancer growth. Genestein also blocks the development of new blood vessels in tumors. Flaxseed contains another isoflavone called lignan, which is rich in omega-3 essential fatty acids, and may have anticarcinogenic effects, may lower LDL, and prevent bone loss.[4]

The recommended daily intake of isoflavones is 30 to 50 mg per day. A higher dose may be harmful. Dr. Susan Love suggests that eating too much may produce a lot of gas. Other side effects of phytoestrogens include vaginal bleeding, depression, and mood swings.

Table 11-a		
Foods with Isoflavones	**Serving**	**Isoflavones (mg)** (approximate values)
Roasted soy nuts	¼ cup dry	62
Tempeh	½ cup	35
Low-fat yogurt	½ cup	35
Regular yogurt	½ cup	35
Regular soy milk	1 cup	30
Low-fat soy milk	1 cup	20
Roasted soy butter	2 tbsp	17
Miso	1 tsp	6
Tofu	4 oz	10
Textured soy protein	½ cup	11
Soy flour	¼ cup	16

Foods Rich in Soy

Tofu is made by adding a curdling agent to soy milk, then pressing the curd into cubes. Phytoestrogens are found in these foods: alfalfa, anise, apples, barley, bluegrass, carrots, cherries, coffee, fennel, licorice, oats, palmetto, parsley, peas, pomegranates, potatoes, grape seeds, red beans, rye, sage, soybeans, corn, chick peas, rice, date palms, and wheat.

Soy and your health: Preliminary research, presented at the American Osteopathic Association, documented that tofu and other soy-based foods (and possibly ginseng) may help women reduce their risk of breast cancer.

Hot flashes were reduced by 47 percent among participants in a randomized placebo-controlled crossover study. Among 51 subjects who took 20 g per day of isolated soy protein for six months, a significant reduction in the recurrence of hot flashes was realized.

A meta-analysis of 38 clinical studies showed an increase in HDL and a decrease in total cholesterol, LDL, and triglycerides in those consuming about 50 g of soy per day.

Soy foods may also increase bone density in postmenopausal women.

Societies with a high soy-product intake typically experience a lower incidence of certain cancers. Soy products reduce the incidence of breast, prostate, and colon cancer; and other cancers such as leukemia and lymphoma.

To increase soy in your diet, when baking, replace one-fourth of the flour required with soy flour. Buy dry roasted soy nuts for snacking. Use miso in soup, and use tofu and tempeh as meat substitutes.

Buyer beware: The isoflavone content of a product greatly depends upon how it is processed. Water extraction results in a high content, while with ethanol extraction, most isoflavones are washed away. You still have a soy product, but without the isoflavones. Be aware that just because it says "soy," it does not mean that isoflavones are present. Some common examples are soy sauce, soybean oil, soy hot dogs, soy cheese, tofu yogurt, and soy bacon—all of which contain a small amount of soy. Some soy products, such as vegetarian or soy burgers, are made with "soy-protein concentrate," which contains almost no isoflavones. Look for products that say "soy-protein isolate" on the label; the isoflavones are largely retained.

Vitamins and Other Supplements

When a woman asks me about vitamins and supplements, my answer always depends upon her eating habits, lifestyle, genetic makeup, and state of health. Ideally, we should get all of the vitamins and minerals we need from our diet. This is not possible for most women, especially menopausal women who require more of certain nutrients to prevent bone loss and heart disease. How much do you personally need? Only you have the answer. Keep a diary of your dietary intake for one week to find out how close you are to the recommended daily doses, and supplement only as needed.

The following supplements confer multiple health benefits, but are specifically good for bone health.

Boron—found in broccoli, beans, cabbage, celery, figs, peaches, plums, parsley, apples, asparagus, and dried fruits (apples, pears, prunes, and raisins). Boron aids the hydroxylation of estrone and estradiol to estriol, and increases the production of estriol. The recommended dosage is 3 mg per day.

Chromium—found in beans, brewer's yeast, brown rice, beer, cheese, wheat grain, whole grain, black cohosh, and red star clover. Chromium helps reduce cholesterol. The recommended dosage is 100 mcg per day.

Copper—found in beans, bittersweet chocolate, nuts, organically grown grains, seafood, and herbs such as skullcap and sage. Copper is necessary for muscle and bone strength and helps decrease cholesterol levels. Copper absorption and utilization can be affected by too much zinc. The recommended dosage is 2 mg per day.

Folic acid—found in leafy green vegetables, wheat germ, and brewer's yeast. Folic acid helps prevent heart disease and maintains an efficient immune system. Alcohol interferes with folic acid absorption. The recommended dosage is 800 mcg per day.

Magnesium—found in cereals, nuts, dark green vegetables, seafood, and animal foods. Magnesium is necessary for calcium absorption, and low magnesium levels can cause vitamin D resistance. Your calcium/magnesium ratio should be 2 to 1. The recommended dosage is 300 to 600 mg per day. Side effects from higher dosages include diarrhea.

Manganese—found in green leaves, seeds, raspberry leaves, ginseng, wild yams, brown rice, and nettles. Manganese is beneficial for conditions such as arthritis, diabetes, and cardiovascular disease. The recommended dosage is 2.5 to 10 mg per day.

Zinc—found in oysters, nettles, pumpkin seeds, spirulina, wild yams, legumes, and whole grains. It is essential for normal bone formation and enhances the action of vitamin D. Zinc also helps keep the immune system in good condition. The recommended dosage is 15 to 50 mg per day. Too much zinc can interfere with copper absorption and utilization.

Vitamin K—found in green leafy vegetables, it is needed to form certain proteins essential for blood clotting, kidney function, and bone metabolism. The recommended dosage is 150 to 500 mcg per day.

Vitamin B_6—found in beef, fish, chicken, bananas, watermelon, and whole grains. Vitamin B_6 has a well-known beneficial effect on PMS and heart disease. The recommended dosage is 25 mg per day. High doses cause neural toxicity.

Other Supplements

DHEA: DHEA (dehydroepiandosterone) is a hormone produced by the adrenal gland. DHEA levels decline with age, dropping by 2 percent per year until death.

Some studies have revealed that DHEA does little more than enhance a feeling of "well-being" at a rate higher than a placebo. In large randomized clinical trials, none of the alleged benefits have been demonstrated.

If you want to try DHEA, the recommended daily dosage is 5 to 10 mg, twice per day. DHEA can be potentially toxic to the liver. Other side effects include breast tenderness, weight gain, hair loss, headache, vertigo, and increased perspiration. Large doses have been associated with muscular development, voice deepening, and clitoral enlargement. Those taking more than 25 mg twice per day should have their liver function, lipid profile, and testosterone levels monitored closely. Women who are trying to lower their estrogen intake should not take DHEA.

Co-enzyme Q_{10} (CoQ_{10}): Co-enzyme Q_{10} (CoQ_{10}) is a cellular constituent involved in energy production. Possible benefits have been seen among individuals with chronic fatigue syndrome, persons with AIDS, in the prevention of heart disease, and in the strengthening of nerve sheaths. The recommended dosage is 30 mg, two to three times per day.

Vitamins and minerals for the perimenopausal and menopausal woman: To achieve the proper levels of vitamins and minerals, supplements are often necessary. The following are RDA recommended doses, as well as the therapeutic dosages of those considered most important.

Table 11-b			
Nutrients	**RDA Recommendation**	**Daily Supplement Range**	**Toxicity Levels**
Beta carotene (Pro Vit A)	10,000–50,000 IU		
Vitamin A	5,000 IU	5,000–10,000 IU	100,000 IU
Vitamin B_1 (thiamine)	1.4 mg	1.1–100 mg	
Vitamin B_2 (riboflavin)	1.4 mg	1.6–50 mg	
Vitamin B_3 (niacinamide)	19 mg	20–100 mg	2,000 mg
Vitamin B_5 (pantothenic acid)	4–7 mg	5–200 mg	
Vitamin B_6 (pyridoxine)	2 mg	4–50 mg	200 mg

Nutrients	RDA Recommendation	Daily Supplement Range	Toxicity Levels
Vitamin B$_7$ (biotin)	150–300 mcg	300 mcg	
Vitamin B$_{12}$ (cobalamine)	3–4 mcg	2.2 to 200 mcg	
Bioflavonoids	500 mg	500–2,000 mg	
Boron*	3 mg		
Bromelain*	100 mg		
Vitamin C	60 mg	70–5,000 mg	
Calcium	800–1200 mg	800–2000 mg	3,000 mg
Choline*	50–100 mg		
Chromium	50–200 mcg	200–500 mcg	200–600 mcg
Copper	2 to 3 mg	2 to 3 mg	
Vitamin D	400 IU	400–800 IU	1,000 IU
Vitamin E (d-alpha tocopherol)	25 IU	200–800 IU	3,000 IU
Folic acid	200 mcg	200–800 mcg	
Inositol*	50–100 mg		
Iodine	150 mcg	50–175 mcg	1,000 mcg

Nutrients	RDA Recommen- dation	Daily Supplement Range	Toxicity Levels
Iron	18 mg	18–30 mg	100 mg
Fluoride*	1.5–4 mg		8,000 mg
Vitamin K	70 mcg	65–500 mcg	
Magnesium	300 mg	300 mg	
Manganese	2.5–5.0 mg	2.5 –10 mg	
Papain*	65 mg		
Para- aminobenzoic acid*	50 mg		
Phosphorus	900–1,200 mg	800–1,200 mg	
Potassium (aspartate)*	1,500–2,000 mg		1,800–5,000 mg
Selenium	55–200 mcg	25–400 mcg	1,000 mcg
Zinc	15 mg	15–50 mg	2,000 mg

* No RDA established

CHAPTER 12

Calcium and Your Health

Throughout life, the body needs calcium to make strong, dense bones and to enable the heart, muscles, and nervous system to work properly. Adequate calcium intake is necessary in childhood and youth for normal bone growth. The average American diet, even a healthy one, may not give you the amount of calcium you need. It has been estimated that the average person consumes about 650 mg of calcium per day.

Table 12-a
NATIONAL INSTITUTES OF HEALTH (NIH) PANEL
CALCIUM RECOMMENDATION PER DAY

Children and Young Adults:

Age 1–10 :	800–1,200 mg
Age 11–24:	1,200–1,500 mg

Adult Female:

Age 25–50:	1,000 mg
Age 50–65:	1,500 mg
Postmenopausal and taking estrogen:	1,000 mg
Pregnant or nursing:	1,200–1,500 mg
Age 65+:	1,500 mg

Your diet should be the first choice for increasing your calcium intake, such as eating leafy green vegetables and legumes, plus calcium-fortified products. Your own food can be fortified by adding a tablespoon or two of nonfat dry milk to baked goods, hot beverages, or casseroles.

Dairy products such as milk, yogurt, and cheese not only contain calcium, but are also a major source of vitamin D; additionally they contain vitamins A, B_6, folate, riboflavin, magnesium, and potassium. Other foods such as broccoli, turnip greens, and canned salmon with bones are also great sources of calcium. It's important to remember that the more protein you consume, the greater your need for calcium. Also, cutting back on daily sodium intake helps to reduce bone loss. An Australian study revealed that postmenopausal women who consume more than 2,100 mg of sodium per day had significantly greater bone loss. When this amount was decreased to less than 2,000 mg a day, it had the same effect as increasing calcium intake by 1,000 mg.[1]

During prolonged immobilization, we have a tendency to lose bone mass. In the event you'll be bedridden for more than a week, you will need to boost your calcium intake up to 2,000 mg a day for about seven times the length of time you are confined. You should also know that taking excess calcium can cause constipation.

Table 12-b
HIGH-CALCIUM FOODS

Food products	Serving size	Calcium/mg
Yogurt		
Low-fat plain	8 oz	450
Low-fat fruit	8 oz	314
Fat-free plain	8 oz	415
Milk		
Whole	8 oz	288
1%	8 oz	300
2%	8 oz	297
Skim	8 oz	302
Powdered nonfat dry milk	1 tsp	50

Cheese

Swiss cheese	1 oz	260
American cheese	1 oz	130
Cheddar cheese	1 oz	204
Cottage cheese		
(1% low fat)	¹/₂ cup	75
Parmesan cheese	1 tbsp	70
Muenster	1 oz	203
Ricotta, part skim	¹/₂ cup	337
Ricotta, whole milk	¹/₂ cup	257

Ice cream

Vanilla, 10% fat	1 cup	175
Vanilla, 16% fat	1 cup	150
Vanilla ice milk, hard	1 cup	175
Vanilla ice milk, soft	1 cup	275

Custard, baked   1 cup   297

Pudding

Chocolate	1 cup	250
Vanilla	1 cup	258

Other Foods

Orange juice, calcium fortified	1 cup	300
Citrus punch with CCM*	1 cup	300
Fruit punch with CCM*	1 cup	300
Molasses, blackstrap	1 tbsp	137
Dried uncooked apricots	1 cup	100
Farina cooked	1 cup	147

Green Leafy Vegetables (cooked unless specified)

Broccoli, fresh	1 cup	175
Broccoli, frozen	1 cup	95
Collard greens	1 cup	300
Mustard greens	1 cup	193
Spinach	¹/₂ cup	122
Chinese cabbage (pak-choi)	¹/₂ cup	79
Kale	1 cup	179
Rhubarb	1 cup	348

Meat, Poultry and Seafood

Salmon (canned with bones)	3 oz	170
Sardines (in oil with bones)	3 oz	370
Oysters, raw	1 cup	226
Eggs	1 medium	55

Beans and Legumes

Soybeans, mature, boiled	1 cup	175
Garbanzo beans, cooked	1 cup	150
Black beans, cooked	1 cup	135
Pinto beans, cooked	1 cup	128
Corn tortilla	2	120

Nuts and Seeds

Sesame seeds	3 tbsp	300
Almonds	1 cup	300
Brazil nuts	1 cup	260
Hazelnuts	1 cup	282
Sunflower seeds	1 cup	174
Walnuts	¹/₂ cup	50
Pecans	¹/₂ cup	42
Tempeh	4 oz	172
Tofu	¹/₂ cup	258

---

*CCM = Calcium citrate-malate

Selecting a Calcium Supplement

Calcium supplements should be an option only if you cannot, or are unwilling to, consume enough calcium as part of your daily diet. If you need a supplement, calcium is available as various salts such as phosphate, citrate, asporotate, and carbonate. It has been recommended that you avoid calcium supplements made from bone meal and dolomite because of the risk of contamination with arsenic, lead, or mercury. Calcium carbonate is the least expensive and provides the highest percentage of available calcium, calcium phosphate is the least likely to cause constipation, and calcium citrate is the most easily absorbed.[2]

Calcium should not be obtained from antacids such as Tums or Rolaids. Antacids decrease the amount of hydrochloride acid in your stomach. Hydrochloride acid is necessary for calcium absorption.[3] By decreasing acidity, absorption is reduced.[4] Over one-third of postmenopausal women have stomach acid deficiency. Taking antacids can reduce calcium absorption from 22 percent to about 4 percent.

How much calcium supplementation do you need? Keep track of calcium intake in your diet for one week, then divide the number by seven to determine your average daily intake. Take calcium supplements for the amount you are lacking.

Some calcium supplements are manufactured in a way that prevents them from breaking down in the gastrointestinal tract. To make sure that your calcium supplement does break down properly, drop one in a glass of vinegar. If it has not broken down in 30 minutes, switch to another brand.

Calcium and magnesium intakes should be balanced. No studies have been done to determine the optional balance; however, 2 mg of calcium for 1 mg of magnesium has been recommended.

Calcium and vitamin D: Vitamin D helps the body absorb and retain calcium. Vitamin D can be obtained via a vitamin D supplement 400 IU daily, through 15 minutes of sun exposure per day, or by consuming certain foods, such as fortified dairy products, eggs, and oily fish such as salmon. Eight ounces of milk contains 100 IU of vitamin D. The recommended dietary allowance of vitamin D is 200–400 IU per day.

Table 12-c
SUPPLEMENTAL SOURCES OF CALCIUM
How Much Calcium Are You Really Getting in a Supplement?

Calcium in supplement	Calcium per tablet(mg)	No. of tablets needed to provide 500 mg of calcium
Calcium carbonate		
Generic USP	500	1
Caltrate	500	1
Biocal	500	1
Tums	200	2.5
Tums E-X	300	1.5
OsCal 500 (chewable)	500	1
Calcium citrate		
Citrical	200	3
Calcium gluconate USP		
generic (Roxane)	45	12
generic (Upjohn)	87.75	6
Calcium lactate USP		
generic (Lilly)	84.5	6

Guidelines for taking a calcium supplement:

• It is best to take calcium (especially calcium carbonate) with food and at night. Absorption increases if calcium is consumed with meals or snacks.

• For better absorption, limit the amount to no more than 600 mg of elemental (available) calcium at one time.

- Calcium should be taken in divided amounts. The body's ability to efficiently absorb calcium drops when it is taken in one big lump rather than in smaller amounts twice a day.

- If your supplement does not contain vitamin D, add a multivitamin with at least 200 to 400 IU of vitamin D.

- Calcium citrate is preferred for women over 60.

Other fringe benefits of calcium: Not only does calcium help protect your bones, some experts believe that it may help the cardiovascular system. Decreased calcium intake has been associated with increased blood pressure, leaving one at risk for heart attack, strokes, and kidney failure. One study demonstrated that a diet rich in calcium lowers blood pressure. Calcium appears to increase the production of nitric oxide, a substance that helps relax and open up blood vessels, thereby reducing blood pressure. However, it was noted that calcium supplements only produced half that increase when compared with a calcium-rich diet. Calcium-rich foods and dairy products also contain potassium and magnesium, which together with calcium, help keep blood pressure in check. Taking calcium supplements has also been associated with a decreased risk of colon cancer.

CHAPTER 13

You and Your Weight

"None of the conventional approaches to losing weight are effective—
in other words, most diets don't work."
— National Institutes of Health

Your body needs a certain amount of calories to function properly. If you ingest too many calories without enough expenditure, the result will be an accumulation of fat in your body—that is, you will be overweight. More than half of the United States adult population and nearly one-fifth of its children and adolescents are overweight.

The percentage of Americans who are obese is climbing at an alarming rate. Obesity is defined as weighing more than 20 percent over ideal body weight. Obesity-related conditions are second only to smoking as leading causes of preventable deaths. If you are overweight or obese, you need to lose weight if you want to avoid the complications related to obesity.

Health Complications of Obesity

Obesity has been found to contribute to death rates from a variety of causes, and is also a factor in the following conditions:

- As many as 80 percent of individuals with Type 2 diabetes are obese.[1]

- High blood pressure, the leading cause of heart disease and stroke, is three times more common among overweight adults than among non-overweight adults.[2]

- High cholesterol, high blood pressure, and diabetes, the major risk factors for heart disease, are all linked to excess weight. They are 1.5 times more common among overweight people than among normal weight people. Obese individuals are twice as likely to develop cancer of the colon, prostate, breast, and uterus. Obesity accelerates osteoarthritis of the hips, knees, and ankles by placing added pressure on joints already damaged.[3]

- Obese individuals are three times more likely to suffer a heart attack than individuals of average weight.[4]

- Obese individuals are more likely to suffer from sleep apnea, a dangerous condition where breathing is continually halted during sleep.

- Obesity is responsible for 53 percent of gallstones.

Causes of Obesity

Obesity is partly inherited and partly environmental. Obese parents generally have obese children. Twins tend to gain weight at the same rate, and the weight is distributed at the same body sites, regardless of whether they are raised together.

The way the body burns calories at rest is called the "resting metabolism." Some women have a slower metabolic rate than others. With aging, a woman's metabolism slows about 0.5 percent per year.

Your weight also depends on your physical activity level. The more you exercise, the higher your metabolic rate and the more calories you burn. Hormonal imbalances, such as an underactive thyroid, lower the metabolic rate.

There are many other factors that influence your weight. People under stress or who are depressed have a tendency to overeat. Antidepressants, and corticosteroids that are taken to treat asthma or rheumatoid arthritis, can cause weight gain. If you were once rather active and have become sedentary, you will no doubt gain weight.

A PERSONAL STORY

It is ironic that I find myself, like everyone else, trying to lose weight. I grew up in a culture where being plump was equated with wealth and health. Women who could afford to injected themselves with "Durabolin," a very expensive steroid, to maintain plumpness.

I remember being self-conscious about my lanky body during my teenage years. Not only did I have to deal with being tall, I was very skinny. My little brother, Lesly, used to call me Gran'Pele, a witch character in our stories who dressed in black and flew on a broomstick. When I was 17, my cousin, Marie Jose, sent me a pair of blue jeans from New York, where she was attending college. It was not customary for girls to wear pants at that time in Haiti. The first and last time I wore those pants, people on the street looked at me as if I were some kind of a freak. One man even asked me if my parents had enough food to feed me!

While I was in medical school, my roommate, Nicole, and I decided that we needed to gain some weight. Nicole was not as tall as I was, but she was obsessed about her belly being too flat. We would save our money and buy fattening food at the cafeteria. From time to time, she would lift up her blouse for me to inspect her belly to see if it was getting any fatter. I used to laugh at her and tell her to eat even more. Today, Nicole is married to another Haitian doctor, Fanell, and has two children, Philip, my godson, and Michele. The years have gone by. We can afford to buy any food we want, but now we are watching our weight. Nicole now complains that her belly is too big, and she wants to lose it. She has become as concerned now about losing weight as she once was about gaining weight.

Are You Overweight or Obese?

Women naturally have more body fat than men. Starting at puberty, estrogen causes females to add fat, particularly in the hips and thighs.

There are two different ways to find out if you are overweight. One is to weigh yourself and compare your body weight to the following chart. The other way is to calculate your body mass index (BMI).

Table 13-a		
USDA SUGGESTED WEIGHTS FOR ADULTS		
Weight in lbs (without clothes)		
Height Without Shoes	Age 19–34	Over 35
5'0"	97–128	108–138
5'1"	101–132	111–143
5'2"	104–137	115–148
5'3"	107–141	119–152
5'4"	111–146	122–157
5'5"	114–150	126–162
5'6"	118–155	130–167
5'7"	121–160	134–172
5'8"	125–164	138–178
5'9"	129–169	142–183
5'10"	132–174	146–188
5'11"	136–179	151–194
6'0"	140–184	155–199

The lower weights usually apply to women who have less muscle and bone. Weight of 5–20 percent over the normal is considered "overweight." Greater than 20 percent above normal is considered "obese."

✣ ✣ ✣

The preceding chart, however, can be misleading. Different women have different bone structures and bone mass. Black women have a higher bone mass than white or Asian women. When I look at myself, I feel very comfortable with my weight and appearance. At six feet tall, my weight fluctuates around 210 pounds. According to the above chart, I am overweight. While I am writing this, my friend Laurie sits next to me. She is

5'3" tall, white, and weighs 107 pounds. According to the chart, Laurie's weight is perfect; however, Laurie looks and feels "skinny." Laurie tells me that when she looks in the mirror, she sees her bones and her ribs and would like a little more padding here and there. (Of course I feel like choking her while she is telling me this!)

When I ask a patient or friend to guess how much I weigh, they always guess between 150 and 160 pounds (I wish!). The only person who thinks that I should lose some weight is my Haitian husband, Albert. He says that I should lose a little more of my belly. Although I wish that my belly could be flatter, I am too much of a coward to consider liposuction. So, I just look at my reflection in the mirror and repeat, "I love and accept everything about my body." (I am learning from Louise Hay.) I have warned Albert that I do not want him to touch my belly—or tell me how fat it is. The only time he can touch it is to give me pleasure; otherwise, he can keep his hands off!

Experts are agreeing that the tables of "ideal weight" are too low. Seriously overweight women have little hope to reach them and will consider themselves a failure. This is why many health-care providers are now relying on the body mass index (BMI). It is a better reflection of body composition and also correlates better with body fat and the risk of obesity-related disease.

It is difficult to evaluate the percentage of body fat. The BMI, on the other hand, is based on information readily available, such as your weight and height. Except for those people whose bodies are obviously mostly muscle, like weight lifters, the BMI is a good indicator of health problems that are related to obesity.

Calculating Your Body Mass Index (BMI)

Calculate your BMI by using the following formula:

Weight (in kilograms)
divided by your
Height (in meters) squared

To convert your weight to kilograms, multiply your weight in pounds by 0.45. To convert your height to meters, multiply your height in inches by 0.0254. For example 140 pounds is equal to 63 kilograms (140 x .45), and

70 inches tall is equivalent to 1.78 meters (70 x .0254). You then square this number (1.782), which in our example equals 3.17. Your BMI can be calculated by dividing your weight of 63 kg by 3.17, which equals 19.87.

$$\frac{140 \times .45}{70 \times .0254 = 1.782 \text{ (squared)}} \quad \frac{= \quad 63}{= \quad 3.17} \quad = \quad 19.87$$

Table 13-b
BMI CHART

BMI no.:	25	26	27	28	29	30	31	32	33	34	35	40
Height					**(Weight in lbs)**							
4'10"	119	124	129	134	138	143	149	153	158	163	167	191
4'11"	124	128	133	138	143	148	154	158	164	169	173	198
5'0	128	133	138	143	148	153	159	164	169	175	179	204
5'1"	132	137	143	148	153	158	165	169	175	180	185	211
5'2"	136	142	147	153	158	164	170	175	181	186	191	218
5'3"	141	146	152	158	163	169	175	181	187	192	197	225
5'4"	145	151	157	163	169	174	181	187	193	199	204	232
5'5"	150	156	162	168	174	180	187	193	199	205	210	240
5'6"	155	161	167	173	179	186	192	199	206	211	216	247
5'7"	159	166	172	178	185	191	198	205	211	218	223	255
5'8"	164	171	177	184	190	197	204	211	218	224	230	262
5'9"	169	176	182	189	196	203	210	217	224	231	236	270
5'10"	174	181	188	195	202	207	216	223	230	237	243	278
5'11"	179	186	193	200	208	215	222	230	237	244	250	286
6'0	184	191	199	206	213	221	228	236	244	251	258	294
6'1"	189	197	204	212	219	227	236	243	251	258	265	302
6'2"	194	202	210	218	225	233	241	250	258	265	272	311
6'3"	200	208	216	224	232	240	248	256	264	272	279	319

A BMI between 19 and 25 is considered normal, between 26 and 30 is considered overweight, and over 30 is considered obese.

How to Lose Weight in a Healthy Manner

Too many women perceive dieting as something that they have to do for only a certain period of time and then they can return to their old habits. This is why statistics show that only 5 to 10 percent of dieters are able to maintain their weight loss after two years.

Successful weight control involves a combination of changes in the amount and type of food eaten, changes in exercise level, and behavior modification therapy. In many cases, the help of a physician, personal trainer, or a nutritionist is necessary.

There is an increased likelihood of success when there is a realistic goal for an outcome, realistic time frames for change, and a realistic commitment to long-term maintenance once change is initiated. You should also realize that weight loss amounts as small as 5 to 10 percent of body weight will impact your health in a positive way.

Everyone has a difficult time changing habits they've had all their lives. Do you want to change the way you eat and the amount you weigh? The important thing is to make up your mind to change; and take small, manageable steps that will help you attain your goal. The old adage "one day at a time" is very applicable here. Losing weight can be difficult, as most social activities involve eating!

For a weight-loss program to be successful, it has to also include an exercise program. Dieting alone is insufficient and contributes to the loss of both muscle and fat.[5]

Losing Weight with Your Doctor's Help

Working with your health-care provider to tailor a diet for your specific health needs is the ideal way to lose weight. Every person is different: Some women are obese because they do not exercise, others because they have a diet consisting of refined sugars and simple carbohydrates. A diet that works for a spouse or a friend may not work for you. Certain medications such as allergy pills, high blood pressure drugs, and antidepressants can affect your weight by slowing your metabolism, increasing your appetite, or making your body retain water. Endocrine disorders such as hypothyroidism (low thyroid) can cause weight gain by slowing metabolism. (This ailment can be ruled out with a simple blood test.)

A good weight-loss program should include screening for medical conditions that may cause weight gain; as well as for depression, stress, anxiety, and eating disorders.

Consult with your health-care provider regarding any over the-counter medications or prescription drugs for weight loss.

Commercial Diet Plans

Commercial diet plans can be deceiving. There is only a 20 percent success rate among weight-loss programs. Ask a trusted health-care provider if the program is sound and appropriate. Remember, programs promising results without dieting and exercise won't work. *There is no such thing as a calorie-free lunch!*

A PERSONAL DIET STORY

Awhile ago, after I had gained some extra weight, I worked hard to lose it once again. I loved how I felt and how I looked in the mirror. I was proud to wear my good clothes that had been waiting patiently in the back of my closet. I remember the first day I was able to wear a beautiful red pantsuit with white trim and gold buttons that my mother had sent me for motivation. I promised myself that I would never gain back that weight. When that red pantsuit began getting too tight, it was a wake-up call! I realized that I was returning to some of my old, unhealthy eating habits.

For example, I remembered that the previous weekend, I had been working very long hours. At the hospital all night and all morning, two days before my period started, I was cranky and hungry. When I got to the hospital cafeteria, the food looked unappetizing. I reluctantly ended up with a piece of chicken and some vegetables. When I got to the cashier, however, I noticed some heart-shaped, milk chocolate candies. I could not control myself! I opened my hand and grabbed as many as I could; eight of them fit in my fist. I started to eat one before I had even paid the cashier.

"Dr. Jean-Murat, I can see that you are hooked on chocolate," the cashier said with a smile. I answered her with a grin, too busy chewing. I then hurried to the corner of the cafeteria, far away from everybody. I did not dare to sit in the small doctor's lounge; I would have been ashamed to be seen.

By the time I had finished the tasteless chicken, I had already eaten four more of the chocolates. I ate two more on the way to my car. More guilt crept over me. *I will save the last one for tomorrow,* I promised myself.

When I got home, the cravings started again, I wanted to eat that last one. Meanwhile, the guilt level was very high, but I didn't care. It was a hot day, and when I tried to unwrap the piece of chocolate, it had melted and was stuck to the foil. I did not want to lose any of the chocolate, but I was a little too ashamed to lick it off. I put it in the freezer and anxiously checked on it until, after what seemed an eternity, the foil could be removed from the intact piece of chocolate. I almost swallowed it whole. Guilt crushed down on me. *I will exercise a lot more, tomorrow,* I told myself, thinking wistfully of my red pantsuit.

❦ ❦ ❦

Here in the U.S., we constantly live with guilt about eating. Most of us are on some kind of diet. What good is it to be able to afford to buy whatever we want when we are restricted because we're trying to lose weight? I have always wondered which is worse: not having enough money to buy food and going hungry, or having all the food we want and sometimes starving ourselves. The solution is that we must eat in moderation. When I go to a restaurant or I am at one of my Haitian friend's homes or my mother's house, I practice moderation by taking a small taste of everything. I realize that if I don't, I will cheat later on. I try to convince myself that this is all I really want! I do not consider this dieting; I see it as doing the right thing.

So, if you're like me, and you have overindulged, or failed to exercise as planned, do not become consumed with guilt or you will soon become discouraged and quit. Instead, enjoy your life, and when you stray, return to your regular schedule with additional moderation as quickly as possible. Guilt only causes you to frown, which causes *wrinkles.*

The Sugar/Carbohydrate Connection

I have learned that if you exercise and watch what you eat, you should be able to lose weight. Most of us, though, are unable to control the amount of food we eat because we are unable to control our cravings. Some people are lucky enough be able to maintain an ideal weight, but eventually, like 60 percent of American adults, we become obese. (For a good book related to this issue, read *Constant Craving,* by Doreen Virtue, Ph.D.)

Time and again, we have heard that to lose weight, we should cut down on fat and eat lots of carbohydrates. Currently, the amount of carbohydrates consumed in an average diet consists of more than two-thirds of our daily food intake. Accordingly, people trying to lose weight are consuming more carbohydrates and cutting down their fat intake.

But according to Morisson C. Bethea, M.D., the author of *Sugar Busters: Cut Sugar to Trim Fat*; Robert C. Atkins, M.D., the author of *Dr. Atkins' New Diet Revolution*; and others, if we could break the sugar habit, we would lose weight and feel great! Insulin, a hormone produced by the pancreas, and weight gain are closely related. The pancreas is a gland located behind the stomach. It secretes the hormones insulin and glucagon that play a role in the regulation of carbohydrate metabolism. The role of insulin is to direct glucose into the cells for immediate needs or to convert glucose so that it can be stored in the muscles and the liver.

It appears that the type and amount of carbohydrates ingested affect the rate of sugar absorption and the release of insulin in the blood. Simple carbohydrates are *quickly* absorbed, resulting in high blood-sugar levels and high amounts of insulin. These carbohydrates have what is called a high glycemic index (HGI). They include table sugar; white flour pastries; ice cream; honey; cakes; molasses; white rice; corn products; white flour pasta; vegetables such as carrots and beets; and fruits such as raisins, pineapple, bananas, and watermelon.

Complex carbohydrates are *slowly* absorbed, resulting in low blood-sugar levels and low amounts of insulin. These carbohydrates have what is called a low glycemic index (LGI). They include fruits such as plums, mangos, apricots, grapes, peaches, and oranges; and unrefined whole or cracked grains, whole-grain pasta and breads, nuts, peas, beans, and sweet potatoes.

Since the body can only store a small amount of glucose at a time, all excess has to be converted to fat in the liver, which is then transported to fat cells for storage. The role of insulin in weight gain is seen through the blocking action of lipase, an enzyme needed for the breakdown of stored fat into fuel. If we would eliminate refined sugar and eat simple carbohydrates in a *limited amount,* our bodies would then go to our stored fat areas when we need the long-term energy to keep going. The result is weight loss. Essentially, what happens is that our craving for refined sugars and simple carbohydrates dissipates, and we consume less calories.

According to Dr. Atkins, if we could limit the amount of carbohydrate intake, we could eat as much fat and protein as we want and still lose weight, maintaining the loss as long as we stick with it. And, those with abnormal lipid profiles will improve their lipid levels.

However, the American diet mostly consists of foods made from refined sugars and simple carbohydrates—they taste good, are readily available, and are very affordable to the average person. The immediate benefit is that they are readily absorbed by the body and used quickly for energy. To put it succinctly, people are simply addicted to sugar. Unfortunately, a few hours after ingesting those high-glycemic carbohydrates, our bodies will be craving more food. And for some of us, we become overweight or obese.

As a doctor, I am usually reluctant to give credence to new theories, especially when they go against everything that I have been taught. How could I recommend to a patient who is obese and who has an abnormal lipid profile that she just quit eating refined sugars and simple carbohydrates and eat a limited amount of complex carbohydrates, eat all the fat and protein she wants, and she would become thin and watch her lipid profile improve!

I had never heard of the sugar/carbohydrate connection with weight loss until my patient Marcy, a 40-year-old who had tried everything to lose weight and improve her lipid profile, remembered that in her 20s, she was overweight, tried the Atkins diet, and kept her weight down—until she went back to her old habits. I was shocked to see Marcy two months later, 15 pounds lighter, with a greatly improved lipid profile and sky-high self-esteem.

As this book goes to print, the jury is still out regarding to whom this diet should be recommended. Would it be the answer for those patients whose obesity is jeopardizing their health? Is it the answer for those who have tried prescription drugs only to find that they are full of side effects? Only time will tell. (Please check my website at **www.drcarolle.com** for updated information and research results.)

❧ ❧ ❧

Watching the scale while trying to lose weight can be disappointing. While losing fat, muscle mass increases, slowing weight loss. Muscle, per unit volume, is approximately twice as heavy as fat! Don't be surprised if your mirror is showing you positive results while your scale is not.

If you are doing your best and not losing weight, don't get discouraged.

Examine the reasons why you're eating. If you are overeating when you're bored, depressed, tired, in crisis, or alone, become aware of these feelings and learn to cope without food. Learning relaxation techniques or getting involved in a new activity for distraction can help take the focus off food.

It's normal for women to gain some weight with aging. Don't beat yourself up if you're no longer the slim size you once were. Exercising regularly is the best way to keep your weight down. Most important, you'll feel good and be healthier.

CHAPTER 14

If You're Sedentary, Learn to Exercise

Exercising regularly is an excellent way to get into good physical condition, and being in good physical condition is synonymous with being in good health. Many studies have demonstrated that if you exercise regularly and eat a balanced low-fat diet, your state of health will greatly improve, as will your ability to prevent certain diseases. Exercise also increases life expectancy.[1] Physical activity significantly decreases the risk of early mortality due to cardiovascular disease, and exercise in postmenopausal women reduces the risk of all causes of mortality.[2]

Unfortunately, six out of ten women lead a sedentary life. They use a car to get around, compete for the parking spaces closest to the store, and take elevators instead of stairs. Many people are "couch potatoes," spending long periods of time in front of the television set or computer. At the same time, they have a high-fat, high-sugar diet and may smoke. This combination is a recipe for fatal heart disease.

Benefits of Regular Exercise

Regular exercise:

- builds strong bones and muscles and reduces the risk of osteoporosis.

- strengthens the heart. It is a major way to decrease the risk of heart disease. Inactive women are three times more likely to die prematurely of a heart attack than active women. Women who walk on a regular basis can decrease their risk of heart disease by 60 to 75 percent. Vigorous exercise cuts the risk of a heart attack in half.

- lowers LDL and raises HDL, preventing atherosclerosis.

- improves the transport and use of oxygen throughout the body.

- reduces the risk of diabetes. Regular exercise lowers the risk of Type 2 diabetes.

- helps diabetics. Obese women store fat in the abdominal area, which increases the resistance of the cells to insulin, making it difficult to control glucose in the blood. Women with diabetes who exercise regularly require less medication to control their disease.

- reduces the risk of hypertension. Consistent aerobic exercise helps prevent high blood pressure and lowers blood pressure. Women who exercise at least 20 minutes a day, three days a week, can control their blood pressure; and women who need medication to control their blood pressure can reduce the need for medication by exercising regularly.

- aids in weight control. By restricting the number of calories eaten each day and exercising regularly, a healthy body weight can be maintained. Exercise increases muscle mass, which in turn, burns more calories during exercise and rest periods.

- lowers the risk of some cancers, such as breast and colon cancer.

- reduces stress. Women who exercise regularly are less likely to suffer from tension, anxiety, and depression, and they generally feel better about life.

- lessens the risk of stroke.

- helps people sleep more soundly.

- can lessen the severity of hot flashes.

- improves the posture.

- builds strong muscles, reducing the risk of falling.

- alleviates stress, which can cause increased cholesterol. It controls weight, which in turn helps bring down the cholesterol count (decreases total cholesterol and increases HDL).

- promotes better digestion and absorption of nutrients.

Your Exercise Plan

Your first step in planning an exercise program should be to consult your health-care provider. The two of you can decide what kind of exercise is best for you and how you should work into it. Ideally, you should check back with your health-care provider periodically to evaluate your improvement.

Before you start any kind of exercise routine, ask yourself these questions:

- What type of exercise should I do?
- How much do I need?
- How long should I do it?
- Do I need specific equipment?
- Will I need special clothing?

Think twice before joining a gym. More than half of the people who do so quit during the first six months. However, if you do so, make sure that it is convenient to your work or home or you won't go.

Most important of all, pick a type of exercise you *enjoy*. Also, ask yourself:

- Do I want to exercise alone or work out with a group?
- What time of day do I want to exercise?

In case you're not sure, try different kinds of exercise and different times of day before making a final choice. Once you decide, stick with your plan. But if you have to choose between varying your workout schedule and skipping a day—vary!

Exercise should be performed on a regular basis at least two or three times a week at the same time for the best results. Plan on 20 to 30 minutes or longer, according to your endurance. Choose a convenient time, and set a specific goal. For example, "Within two months, I will be swimming three times a week for half an hour."

If you've been inactive for a long time, it's dangerous to overdo at the beginning. Start slowly, and gradually increase the length of time. For example, swim for about 15 minutes the first time, and add two to five minutes a day until you reach your goal.

Be careful not to hurt yourself. Older women who exercise too vigorously can hurt themselves. Take some time to warm up by stretching your legs, arms, and upper-body muscles. When you've finished exercising, cool down in the same way. Dress properly, especially if you exercise outdoors. Be sure to drink plenty of fluids, especially during hot weather so you avoid becoming dehydrated.

If you're interested in using exercise machines, make sure you know how to use them properly *before* you start.

Most of all, listen to your body. If you feel any kind of pain, stop. Exercising should be fun and should improve your health—not hurt it! "No pain, no gain" is a fallacy and could be injurious to your body and overall health.

Water exercises: Water exercising is a great way to enjoy the benefits of aerobic exercise without the negative impact of muscle soreness and aching joints, which usually result in flagging motivation! Water exercise is also ideal for people with diminished physical capabilities, those with painful joints (as in the case of arthritis), and those who are recovering from joint surgery. It's also beneficial for people recovering from leg and back surgery, and it's excellent for pregnant women. The temperature of the water should be between 82 to 86 degrees Fahrenheit.

A Personal Story

I didn't realize the benefit of water exercise personally until I broke my right ankle by missing a step. It happened the day after President Clinton missed a step and badly tore up his right knee. My friends made fun of me, saying that I was parroting the president! While Clinton was on his trip to Finland, worrying about his dignity, I was in California worrying about getting on and off the john! I really wanted to send him an e-mail telling him: "Mistah President, ah feel your pain." But my computer was acting up and by the time it got fixed, we were both recovering.

What I missed the most during the recuperation days was my exercise routine: I had been walking 12 miles a week. My appetite did not realize that I was not burning off the calories. No break there! That was when I started to use my pool for exercise. I bought a house with a pool but had been in it only three times since I moved in—and only then because I was thrown into the water during some wild parties!

I recommend water exercise to my patients who are recuperating from surgery or who sustain injuries that preclude their regular exercise routine, so I had to use my own advice! I went to a sporting goods store and bought a special belt, shoes, and weight attire. With them, I could walk in the water, or run or dance as fast as I could. To do it the right way, I read the book *Fantastic Water Workouts,* by MaryBeth Pappas Gaines, and followed her advice. I still use my water workouts from time to time because it's fun and effective.

🌿 🌿 🌿

Personal trainers: If you can afford it, hiring a personal trainer is a great way to motivate yourself to exercise. A few years ago, I was experiencing some severe pain on one side of my mid-back. The pain was exacerbated if I had to use a vacuum extraction to deliver a baby or perform a Cesarean section where the patient had to be placed in the left tilt position (a safe position for the fetus before delivery). The pain was getting worse, so I went to see a colleague, Grady Anderson, an orthopedist. He told me that I just had to do some specific exercises to strengthen my upper back. He referred me to Steve Haynes, a physical therapist and personal trainer.

Steve had me join a gym and would meet me there twice a week for a workout and stretching, and then give me a good massage, all within one hour. I whined and complained the whole time except when I was getting the massage, which was the only thing I liked.

Steve would call me the night before to remind me about our appointment the next day. He was always there waiting for me at the gym. It seemed that I could not escape that man! I worked with him regularly and started to space out the encounters until my back was in good shape. Whenever I feel any tension in my mid-back, I once again start doing the routines Steve taught me until I feel fine again.

Keeping the Momentum Going!

A Personal Story

One Saturday before going out for my daily walk, it started to rain. I was so disappointed. On several previous walking days it had rained as well, so I had used the treadmill instead, but I have tender knees, and when I use the treadmill too often, they get sore. I did not want to cancel my walk again!

"What about using the umbrella to walk?" I asked my walking companion, Laurie. She agreed, and so we went. I laughed as I remembered that when I used to play tennis years ago, I used to pray for rain so I could cancel. I yelled with joy, while making sure I did not slip in the mud, "I am hooked on exercise!" It was a great feeling.

❧ ❧ ❧

Exercise is an essential part of a successful weight-loss plan. It helps burn calories and influences the appetite-regulating center in the brain.

If you want to lose weight, exercise helps in two ways. First, it controls your appetite. Second, it increases your metabolic rate so you burn calories faster.

To lose one pound of weight, you need to burn 3,500 calories! In order to burn fat, you need to find a comfortable workout level that allows you to constantly move the muscles for about 30 minutes. To start losing weight at the rate of one pound per week, you should exercise for at least 45 minutes, four to five times a week. Then, when you reach your desired weight, to keep fit, you can go back to exercising 30 minutes, three times a week.

The following list gives you some ideas for developing your own program. Remember: Set realistic goals such as mine—I'll walk 2.4 miles around the lake on Tuesdays, I'll use my treadmill for 47 minutes on Thursdays, and walk 3.2 miles on Saturdays.

Table 14-a

ACTIVITY	CALORIES BURNED PER HOUR
Aerobics	400
Belly dancing	250–300
Bicycling (slow)	350
(fast)	600–700
Bowling	150
Calisthenics	400
Child care (stooping, bending, lifting, twisting)	300–400
Dancing (slow)	150
(fast)	300
Driving a car	120
Gardening (some lifting, stooping, digging)	200
Golf (using driving cart)	200
(walking)	400
Housework	150–250
Jumping rope (moderate)	400
(fast)	600
Raking yard	250
Reading, studying	100

ACTIVITY	CALORIES BURNED PER HOUR
Running (slow, 6 mph)	700
(fast, 9 mph)	1,000
Sex	200–400
Shoveling (heavy)	600
Skating (ice or roller, fast)	700
Skiing (downhill, fast)	350
Sleeping	80
Stair climbing	800
Swimming (slow)	400
(fast)	750
Tennis	400
Typing	120
Volleyball	400
Walking (fast)	400
Watching TV	100

These are ballpark estimates (for a woman of 125 pounds). Increase the calories by 10 percent for every 15 pounds of body weight above 125.

Remember:

- In order to burn fat, your workout level must allow you to constantly move your muscles for about 30 minutes.

- Stop that huffing and puffing! Burn fat by keeping a steady pace. If you exercise with someone else, work at a rate that allows you to talk to your partner. When you cannot carry on a conversation, you have exceeded the level for fat metabolism, and the muscles will switch from burning fats to carbohydrates for fuel.

- It takes about a month of working out for 30 minutes, three times per week, for the body to learn to use oxygen more efficiently. While exercising, it takes most of us a full ten minutes for our bodies to get in gear, ready to burn those calories.

CHAPTER 15

If You Smoke, You Must Quit

S moking is the single most preventable cause of illness and premature death. Women tend to be heavier smokers, start at younger ages, and are less successful in quitting than men.[1] In addition to cigarettes, small cigars have come into vogue with women smokers.

Black women are more likely to smoke and less likely to quit. Previously, black teenagers were less likely to smoke than their white counterparts. However, since 1996, there has been only a 30 percent increase in white teenage smoking, compared to an 80 percent increase in black teenage smoking.

Smoking and . . .

. . . **Menopause:** Many studies have revealed a close relationship between smoking and an early occurrence of menopause. The median age of menopause is about age 50. Women who smoke start having menopausal symptoms at a median age that is one to two years earlier than age 50. Basically, the more a woman smokes, the earlier she will begin menopause.[2] Women smokers also have a higher rate of bone loss after menopause, which increases their risk of osteoporosis.

. . . **Cancer:** Cigarettes not only contain nicotine, a very addictive drug, but with each puff, a smoker's body is exposed to over 4,000 other chemicals, more than 40 of which are known to cause cancer.

More American women die of lung cancer than from any other type of cancer. By avoiding smoking, a woman can greatly reduce her risk of lung cancer; as well as heart disease, stroke, emphysema, and other forms of chronic lung disease.

Women who smoke also have an increased risk of cervical cancers. The heavier the smoking, the greater the risk.[3]

. . . **Depression:** One study has shown that daily smoking is associated with a significantly increased risk of major depression. Light smokers who are depressed were three times as likely to increase their smoking. Major depression was about twice as likely to develop in heavy smokers, when compared with infrequent smokers. Similar relationships exist between depression and illicit drug use.

. . . **Heart disease:** Smoking is a major risk factor with respect to heart disease. Some new research has shown that arteries of smokers, ex-smokers, and those exposed to secondhand smoke harden much faster than those of nonsmokers, thus increasing the risk of heart attack and stroke. Women smokers decrease their life expectancy by five to eight years.

Secondhand Smoke

Up to 35,000 deaths from heart attacks in the United States each year are thought to be caused by "passive" smoking. Secondhand smoke is responsible for 150,000 to 300,000 ailments in children per year. There is a 30 percent higher risk of lung cancer in women whose spouse is a smoker.

It is your right to ask people around you to refrain from smoking. Do not allow others to smoke in close proximity to you—in the car, in your home, or in enclosed outdoor areas.

MY POINT OF VIEW

I feel lucky that I do not smoke. It was not the thing for a girl to do when I was growing up in Haiti. When patients talk about nicotine cravings, I can only relate it to food cravings. Whenever we have a small earthquake in California, I always fear that I could be stuck in a place where there is no food. My worst nightmare is being abandoned on a small island with one fruitless coconut tree and no drinkable water. When I am hungry, I have to eat. My family, my friends, and my staff know it. Sometimes I am ashamed of times when I have found myself in some corner of the world stopping for fast food due to uncontrollable cravings. So, I do understand the concept of craving something physically, emotionally, and mentally.

I also empathize with those affected by secondhand smoke. I've had environmental allergies since I was a child. Being exposed to any kind of air pollution makes me very ill. It usually starts with an itchy nose, then difficulty breathing, and, if I remain in the environment, it will be followed by an acute headache.

Living in California where anti-smoking sentiments are high has been a haven for my personal health. Since the only close contact I now have with smokers is with my patients, my sensitivity to cigarette smoke is getting worse, but this actually helps my patients.

I have found that one incentive for a woman to quit smoking is the simple fact that it is emphasized by her health-care provider at each visit. An article in the newsletter of the American College of Obstetrics and Gynecology, of which I am a Fellow, stressed that the practitioner should be sure to discuss smoking cessation with each smoker during each visit. This article, along with my allergies, has prompted me to scold my patients without mercy!

I do not have to read the health questionnaire of a new patient or hear from her that she hasn't quit smoking to know if she smokes. I just have to be in close enough proximity to smell her! I have always told patients rather bluntly that they "stink," and because of my allergies, their visit would have to be limited to their current complaint. Unfortunately, patients who smoke cannot linger to chat with me, which I like to do when time permits.

I also tell them that they are inconsiderate, because they come to see me so that they will experience better health, and in the process, they are making me sick! They promise that they will quit before the next visit, often agreeing on a date to quit before leaving my office.

Some of my colleagues cannot believe that I really interact in this way with my patients. It may seem rude to some people, but this approach really seems to work. It is a personal triumph when I have a patient who has been smoking for years tell me that she finally quit because she was tired of hearing me tell her about the "stink." Should I stop telling patients to quit smoking? The patients themselves urge me to continue this practice of "tough love." So, patients who are smokers, watch out!

❦ ❦ ❦

It is amazing that many patients of mine will discuss prescription medications at length, will reject estrogen replacement when indicated because they are afraid of endometrial or breast cancer, and will demand "natural" remedies, but will continue smoking a pack a day.

If you smoke, you must quit. Quitting smoking cuts the risk of heart disease in half within three to five years[4] and increases life expectancy.

Strategies That Can Help You Quit Smoking

I have been told by many of my patients who smoke that attempting to quit is one of the hardest things to do. Many of them managed to quit during pregnancy, only to resume after they gave birth. Some women have relatives with a history of emphysema or lung cancer, and still they smoke.

Cigarettes are highly addictive, but people can still find the courage and willpower to quit if they are motivated. First, you must *want* to quit, then find a way to do so that fits within your lifestyle. Just because you try and fail once or twice does not mean that you will never succeed. You *can* do it. Just keep trying!

Before you quit:

- You can decide to quit cold turkey—a lot of people have done it. I have had many patients over the years who told me that they just quit all of a sudden because they were tired of me telling them how much they "stink."

- You can speak with your health-care provider about smoking-cessation program and/or nicotine replacement products.

- You can set a quit date: "I'll quit in two months. I'll quit on my birthday." Mark on your calendar the date that you have chosen, and stick to it. Many of my patients who quit smoking did so on the day that we both agreed would be best for them.

- Choose a reliable smoking-cessation program—good programs have a 20 to 50 percent success rate. I do not prescribe any medication to a patient until she has set a date and has made an appointment to start such a program. I do not just hand out pills. A patient really has to show me that she is committed.

- List your reasons for quitting: "I am quitting for myself, my family's health; I have promised my health-care provider that I will stop smoking before my next visit."

Change your behavior: Record how many cigarettes you smoke a day, and when. Then try to smoke half as many. Wait at least five minutes before you light up. Do not smoke at home, in your car, or in the presence of other people. With your partner, make a pact to quit smoking if he or she smokes. Write down your pledge and use it as an affirmation.

After you quit:

- Get rid of all ashtrays and lighters, including those in your car.

- Drink plenty of fluids.

- Cut back on caffeine and alcohol.

- After eating, if the urge to smoke is very strong, brush your teeth, use a mouthwash, or go for a walk.

- Find a way to deal with stress, such as meditating or weight training.

- To control the urges, take a deep breath, hold it for two to three seconds, and exhale slowly through your mouth. Repeat two to three times. It's good to remember that the urge will go away whether you smoke or don't smoke.

- Change daily routines as much as possible.

- Socialize with nonsmokers. Some of my patients have confessed that when they stopped smoking, they also had to make new friends (like those who lose a lot of weight or stop drinking alcohol).

- Avoid visiting places where smoking is prevalent.

- You may gain some weight when you quit smoking because of the oral fixation. Munch on low-calorie vegetables, and keep other low-calorie snacks handy. Exercise helps relieve the urge to smoke and helps you lose those unwanted pounds.

- Make a list of reasons of why you want to quit, and frequently read them.

The first week after quitting is the toughest; but don't worry—it will get better as time goes on!

Other Techniques for Quitting

One interesting "be smoke-free in 21 days" technique was published in the *Journal of Consulting and Clinical Psychology*. The technique is as follows: Count the number of cigarettes you usually smoke in one day. Let's say it's one pack a day, or 24. Cut that number by one-third, down to 16. The key is to smoke those 16 cigarettes at evenly spaced intervals, or one for each waking hour. The second week, divide the original number by three, which equals eight, then smoke one cigarette every two hours. The third week, smoke one-third fewer cigarettes than you did the first week, and continue to cut a third of this number every other day until you are down to one or two cigarettes a day.

Other techniques include hypnosis and acupuncture, especially for heavy smokers—those who smoke two or more packs daily.

Hydrotherapy: It has been suggested by John A. Sherman, N.D., of Portland, Oregon, that taking an Epsom salt bath helps pull nicotine and tar from the skin to prevent its introduction into the bloodstream. Use half a pound of epsom salt per bath. Afterwards, shower or bathe with regular water, and pat the body dry with a towel.

Aversion therapy: Here is another suggestion from Dr. Sherman: Stop smoking for all but one hour a day. During that hour, smoke constantly. Take 15 drops of lobelia tincture a half hour before the first cigarette and again 15 minutes before the last cigarette. Take the same amount of the tincture every 15 minutes during the remainder of the smoking hour. This will result in nausea. Its association with smoking can eliminate the desire for cigarettes in just five to six days.

Quitting Smoking and Weight Gain

One reason why women tend to gain weight after they quit is that they have a tendency to replace cigarettes with food. One easy way to ensure that you will not gain weight after you quit smoking is to make sure that you eat a well-balanced diet, including fruits, vegetables, or air-popped popcorn without butter as snacks. You have all heard about those eight glasses of water a day. If you have not been drinking them, start now. Increasing water intake between meals will give you a sensation of fullness. Also, there could not be a better time to start with a regular exercise program. Exercise will not only help you keep your weight down, it will minimize withdrawal symptoms. And if, in spite of all of your efforts, you still gain a few pounds, remember all the good health benefits you have reaped as a result of quitting smoking. So, hang in there.

Of course, quitting smoking does not always mean that you *have* to gain weight. A study recently published in the *New England Journal of Medicine* found that when using the antidepressant Zyban, people stopped smoking successfully with half the typical weight gain.

I suggest that you do not try to quit smoking during the holidays when there is a lot of tempting food around. Also, do not try to quit when you are under a lot of stress.

Using acupuncture may also help you avoid the weight gain associated with quitting.

What You Need to Know about Nicotine Replacement Products

Nicotine replacement products include Nicorette gum and Nicotine patches, which are readily available without a prescription. Nicotine inhalers can be obtained with a prescription from your health-care provider. These products can help you stop smoking by providing your body with nicotine and reducing withdrawal symptoms.

It has been shown that a smoking-cessation program, combined with nicotine replacement products, produces a higher rate of success than either method alone. These programs are designed to give emotional support to smokers, using one-on-one counseling and self-help methods. While smoking-cessation programs alone can be very effective for light smokers, heavy smokers should opt for the combination of the cessation program in conjunction with a nicotine patch, gum, spray, or inhaler. There are many reliable smoking-cessation programs available at local hospitals and at the YWCA. For a program near you, call the American Lung Association at 800-LUNG-USA, or Smokenders at 800-828-4357.

Zyban and smoking cessation: Zyban is now available to help curb the cravings and moderate the withdrawal symptoms that make quitting so difficult, but it contains no nicotine. It has been prescribed as Wellbutrin for depression. Check with your health-care provider if you would like to try it.

Cigar Smoking and Health Risks

Cigar smoking is becoming a popular pastime for both men and women. In the United States, cigar sales have increased by 50 percent since 1993. Young and middle-aged white males, with higher than average incomes and education, are eight times more likely to smoke than females.

Those who smoke cigars should know that this is not as innocuous a habit as they think. According to a recent report from the National Cancer Institute, daily cigar smoking can lead to cancers of the tongue, lip, mouth, throat, larynx, esophagus, and lungs, as well as chronic obstructive pulmonary disease and coronary heart disease.

Inhalation does have a strong effect on disease risks. Daily cigar smokers who reported inhaling deeply had 27 times the risk of oral cancer, 15 times the risk of esophageal cancer, and 53 times the risk of cancer of the larynx when compared to nonsmokers.

Among cigar smokers who do not inhale, there is a seven times greater risk of oral cancer when compared with nonsmokers, and the risk of cancer of the larynx is more than ten times greater.

Cigar smokers also have an increased risk of lung and heart disease when compared to nonsmokers. Those who inhale "slightly" have double the risk of chronic obstructive pulmonary disease, and they increase their risk of coronary heart disease by 23 percent.

When researchers measured the concentration of carbon monoxide at two cigar events in San Francisco, it was higher than the levels found on a busy California freeway.

I strongly believe that smoking is not merely a bad habit—but a powerful addiction. Quitting can be very challenging, but if you really have the desire to quit, you *can* do it!

CHAPTER 16

Alcohol, Drugs, and Your Health

Alcoholism (and its consequences) represents one of the major causes of death in women between 25 and 64 years of age. The physical effects of alcohol abuse include deterioration of brain activities, diminished mental alertness, lack of physical coordination, poor judgment, and an increased possibility of becoming involved in automobile accidents or other calamities, such as falling and fracturing a hip.

Alcohol abuse also leads to an increased incidence of depression, high blood pressure, cirrhosis of the liver, obesity, stroke, and cancer. Alcohol consumption also increases the risk of breast cancer in women and has been associated with hip and forearm fractures in middle-aged women.[1]

Women who abuse alcohol may abuse drugs as well. They also have a tendency to stay in abusive relationships and are more likely to engage in risky sexual behavior. Older women who abuse alcohol can be difficult to detect because they often live alone.

Do You Consume Too Much Alcohol?

You may believe that alcohol can actually be beneficial to your health. But how much alcohol is the right amount? When experts talk about drinking to protect the heart, they tend to agree that the limit is one drink for women and two for men per day. Remember that all drinks are not equal because different beverages contain varying amounts of alcohol. The right amount to qualify for a light drink is as follows: for wine, 5 ounces; beer, a single 12-ounce can or bottle; and hard liquor, 1.5 ounces of 80 proof. One must also remember that a drink does not mean the same for everyone because of differences in body weight, metabolism, and general health.

You probably consume too much alcohol if you can answer yes to any of these questions:

- Do you drink more than two alcoholic drinks a day?

- Do you crave a drink in the morning?

- Has anyone ever commented that you may be drinking too much?

- Do you feel that you have to have a drink at certain times of the day?

- Do you feel you need a drink to settle your nerves?

- When questioned, are you truthful about the amount you drink?

- Do you feel deprived if you don't drink?

- Do you need a designated driver every time you go to a party?

Illegal Drug Abuse

The abuse of prescription drugs can be a significant problem for women during menopause. Women have less of a tendency to abuse illegal drugs than men; however, women abuse prescription drugs more often and frequently do so in combination with alcohol.

African Americans have a higher incidence of drug abuse. It has been speculated that taking drugs is viewed as a way to deal with stress, pain, disappointment, racism, sexism, and abuse. Many times, drugs are used because "it makes a woman feel good," then she gets hooked on that feeling.

Getting Help for Your Addictions

If drinking is becoming a problem in your life, you should seek assistance. Call Alcoholics Anonymous (AA), Al-Anon, or the National Association for Adult Children of Alcoholics; they can provide support and information. Acupuncture can also be helpful in severe recidivist alcoholism.

If you abuse illegal drugs or prescription medications, talk to your health-care provider, or see a counselor who is trained in helping people in your situation.

CHAPTER 17

Sexuality and the Mature Woman

My mother told me, "What I liked the most about menopause was that I didn't have any more periods, there was no more fear of pregnancy, and the sex was better." This has been confirmed by just about all of the postmenopausal Haitian women I've interviewed.

One of my Haitian friends, who is now 82 years old and wishes to remain anonymous, told me that up until the week before her husband's death from a long illness, she made sure that her sex life was satisfactory. After he died, she made soup with okra, hoping that it would cool off her fiery desire, but it didn't work! A friend suggested some tea made with aloe, which worked to some extent. Her only recourse was frequent showers. Her children and grandchildren could not understand why she was taking so many!

This increase in sexual drive is not only experienced by Haitian women. I have met women from different backgrounds and cultures who have had similar sentiments. Some women have described a new relationship after menopause as "the most emotionally and sexually satisfying" of their lives. On the opposite end of the spectrum, some patients equate menopause with aging and may lose interest in sex.

The findings from my research with Haitian women are confirmed by

The Hite Report.[1] Many women acknowledged that their sexual desire increased with age—sex actually got better.

Factors such as cultural background, religious beliefs, socioeconomic status, and availability of partners affect the frequency and quality of a woman's sexual activity. I also believe that some women from various industrialized cultures may experience a decline in their sexuality because they live in a youth-oriented society where they are being bombarded by the message that sex and beauty are equated with youth.

It is a myth that as women grow older they become sexually abstinent.

According to a survey conducted by *Parade* magazine, older women have sex an average of 2.5 times a month. One-third of women over age 65 are still sexually active. Sixteen percent of women older than 65 state that sex is still important to them. Sexually active women are happier with life in general. Sexual difficulties include reduced sex drives and difficulty achieving orgasm; one third of the women surveyed reported being self-conscious during sex.

Sexual Desire

According to Masters and Johnson, sex drive is not related to estrogen and should not automatically decrease at menopause.[2]

Sexual desire has three distinct but interrelated components. The first one is sexual drive, or the biological basis that is related to hormonal levels. Sexual desire is reflected in sexual fantasies and physical manifestations of sexual interest, such as genital tingling. A woman's culture, her energy level, and life experiences determine her sex drive. Sex drive starts to develop during puberty and is controlled by the brain; hence, the saying, "The brain is the sexiest organ of the body!"

Sex drive does not decrease with age, except as a reaction to problems within the environment, a decrease in general health or energy, the lack of a partner, or moral injunctions against masturbation.

The second component of sexual desire is the cognitive aspect: religious beliefs, childhood training, expectations, and values about sexuality. A woman whose children have moved out of the house may find herself enjoying this newfound privacy, and her level of desire may increase. Another woman whose sexual upbringing makes her believe that grandmas should not be sexual may experience a decline in sexual desire with aging.

Marital happiness is of great importance to continued sexual desire.[3]

The third component is motivation, which plays an important role in sexual desire. If a woman is motivated to be sexual, she will act upon it.

A woman's entire body, including her five senses, is involved in sexual desire. With a loving partner, a woman may never lose her desire for sex. During menopause, because the male hormone is diminished, a woman may experience a reduction in sexual desire. Depression, severe illness, hot flashes leading to insomnia and fatigue, being busy pursuing a goal, problems at work, financial crises, marital problems, unsatisfying sex, lack of communication with a partner, and problems with the children or parents can all affect a woman's desire for sex.

A PATIENT'S STORY

Carol, an 80-year-old new patient, explained that she needed help with something quite private; she even got up and made sure that no one was in the hallway and that the door of my office was closed tight. In a whisper, she confided that she wanted to have sex all the time, that something was wrong with her! Carol was a widow who had been married to the same man for more than 55 years. During the ten years prior to his death, he was impotent. About three months before her visit to my office, Carol had a wild fling with a 40-year-old virile man. They broke off shortly afterward, leaving Carol in a predicament. All her male friends were old and married. The few young men she knew were not attracted to her. She felt lost. Carol also explained that her Catholic upbringing, her pride, and the fear of catching a sexually transmitted disease would not allow her to participate in a sexual encounter with a male prostitute. What was she to do?

Carol was hoping that I could give her a pill to diminish her desire. I told her that there was no such pill! Instead, I had a very open discussion with her about masturbation and the use of sexual aids. I told her that there were stores that carried such items, and there were also catalogs available. As Carol was leaving my office, she asked me if she could give me a hug, during which she whispered in my ear: "I'm going to get a wig and dark glasses and then take a trip to one of those stores today!"

Painful Sex

The decrease in the hormonal milieu can cause pain, thus reducing the frequency of sex. A study found that 70 percent of menopausal women had no or negligible vaginal dryness. Among postmenopausal women who are not on hormonal therapy and who engage in coitus infrequently, the vaginal canal may eventually lose its elasticity and become shorter.

On the other hand, estrogen levels may fall during menopause. If a woman has frequent intercourse, however, the vaginal mucosa will remain healthy.[4]

If a woman experiences pain during intercourse due to vaginal atrophy, she may tend to avoid sexual contact. Her partner's fear of hurting her can lead to his own sexual problems, including impotence.

Atrophic vaginal tissues are also more prone to vaginal infection, such as yeast and bacterial infections. The use of lubricants such as K-Y Jelly, Lubrin, vegetable glycerine, Moist Again, Replens, vitamin E oil, and Astroglide keep the vagina healthy and less prone to infection, and makes vaginal penetration more comfortable. Estrogen is the quickest and most effective way to relieve vaginal atrophy. For patients who have no contraindication to using estrogen, I not only place them on an oral or transdermal estrogen regimen, I also have them use Premarin, Estrace, or Estriol vaginal cream every night at bedtime for two weeks, then every other night for two weeks. Results have been excellent.

PATIENTS' STORIES

I have a patient, Janice, a 55-year-old woman with an estrogen phobia. Her sex life was almost nonexistent, and her husband, who was younger, was complaining. Janice's vaginal entrance was so small I could barely introduce the smallest speculum. I finally convinced her to use the vaginal ring Estring. I showed her a copy of the article that indicated that the estrogen in Estring is barely absorbed systemically. I told her that by the time 90 days was over, her vagina would be healthy, and that resuming an active sex life would keep it healthy. She could also use lubrication, vitamin E oil, and consume flaxseed oil along with a diet enriched with soy products. Janice finally agreed, with great results.

Another patient, Carolyn, came to see me two years after menopause with severe vaginal atrophy, which prevented intercourse. Carolyn had been trying what she called "natural treatments," which did not work. Her husband, a chiropractor, was reluctant to let her use any conventional estrogen therapy. I was able to convince Carolyn to use an estrogen and progesterone cream mixed especially for her by a local compound pharmacist. Since she was on her way to a long-awaited vacation to celebrate her 25th anniversary, I advised her to try the vaginal cream, which she did. Two weeks later, I received a postcard from the happy couple thanking me for the advice and telling me that they were having a great time!

Medical Factors That Affect Sexuality

Many medical factors can affect a woman's sex drive. These include chronic illness such as diabetes mellitus or arthritis, heart disease, hypertension, and hypothyroidism—all causing low energy.

Sexuality after a hysterectomy: A hysterectomy can affect sex drive when a woman believes that the uterus equates to her femininity. One study has demonstrated that as many as 25 to 45 percent of women over the age of 45 who had a hysterectomy, with or without the removal of the ovaries, experienced this loss of femininity. Usually, intercourse should be avoided for about four weeks following surgery. Many of my older female patients have requested a prescription, stating that they could not have sex for six months following the surgery. On the other hand, some women cannot wait four weeks to resume intercourse.

Following a hysterectomy, there may be a change of sensation during intercourse and orgasm, but this change can be minimal and should not interfere with sexual function or achieving orgasm. On the contrary, some women who may have had a hysterectomy because of pain or irregular bleeding may find a great improvement in their sex lives when those symptoms are gone.

PATIENTS' STORIES

One month following a vaginal hysterectomy, my patient Judy left a message to have me call her right away. She had followed my advice not to have intercourse for four weeks, and her husband had been complaining almost daily about this lack of intimacy. Judy could not understand this; her husband was in his 50s, and she thought he would have cooled off by now. They were at a restaurant when he realized that the four-week moratorium was over. He said to a startled Judy, "Eat fast, we have to hurry home!" Judy's husband was usually a very careful man when it came to driving, but he drove home exceeding the speed limit. When intercourse was over, he looked very disappointed. "I felt that I was hitting a rock," he said to her.

As Judy explained his reaction, I thought that one of the sutures may have hardened, so I asked her to come in for a look. When I visualized the vaginal vault with the help of a speculum, I saw that it was healing very well. There was only a small remnant of a suture, which was very soft. I told Judy that her husband's experience could be due to the scarring and healing process. Eventually, the abnormal sensation went away, and Judy and her husband now have a satisfying sex life.

Another patient, Sandra, age 41, was finalizing her pre-op paperwork at my office, when suddenly she started to cry. She told me that she did not want to have the surgery. She had a uniformly enlarged uterus with heavy bleeding and severe cramps that were not relieved with the strongest analgesic. I suspected not only fibroids, but also a disease called adenomyosis, when the glands that line the uterus are also present within the body of the uterus, causing severe pain during menses. Sandra confessed that a girlfriend said her sex life would go down the drain following the hysterectomy. Because she and her husband loved to have sex frequently, she was willing to suffer the pain until menopause rather than lose that intimacy.

I explained to Sandra that some women who must lose their ovaries along with the uterus may have some symptoms, but if the right amount of estrogen is taken, there may be no problems. I was not going to remove Sandra's ovaries, so I told her she did not have to worry. Sandra had her hysterectomy, and adenomyosis was found. Whenever I see her now and ask how her sex life is, she happily answers, "Great!"

Sexuality after cancer: A woman's sexuality is usually affected following the diagnosis and treatment of cancer. Breast cancer, particularly after a mastectomy, can have a major psychological effect on both the woman and her partner. About one-third of women have not resumed sexual activity within six months after the mastectomy. A woman's self-esteem may be diminished because she feels deformed, less sexually attractive, and she may also experience rejection from her partner.

Many women who have experienced a mastectomy cope with it as they would with any life-saving surgery. Medical advances in reconstructive surgery and new feminine apparels, have women coping favorably with their changed body.

Sexuality and . . .

. . . **Drugs:** Medications, including recreational drugs and alcohol, are big players in sexual function. Drugs affecting sexual response are high-dose sedatives, antihypertensives, antipsychotic drugs, diuretics, high doses of marijuana and cocaine, and amphetamines.

Drugs used for depression that block testosterone utilization or decrease its synthesis are opiates, SSRI drugs such as fluoxetine (Prozac), and sertraline (Zoloft). Drugs with a less negative effect are Wellbutrin and Serzone.

If you are taking any of these drugs and are having sexual problems, you should check with your health-care provider and discuss the possibility of a "drug holiday." A drug holiday (weekend) consists of stopping the medication on Friday morning and restarting Sunday. However, this may precipitate depression. A drug holiday should only be done when the patient's depressive disorder is relatively stable and well controlled. Another option is switching to another drug.

. . . **Premature menopause:** In a younger woman who has to undergo a hysterectomy and the removal of the uterus and the ovaries, the symptoms of hormonal deficiency, especially that of testosterone, are sometimes severe. This also occurs in women who receive chemotherapy treatments for cancer.

Among younger women with severe endometriosis, the uterus, the tubes, and both ovaries have to be removed. I have had many young women who are in their 30s feel miserable because they are not getting enough estrogen and testosterone. It seems that many health-care providers feel that these patients should be able to do well with the same hormone dosage given to postmenopausal women.

PATIENTS' STORIES

Debra came into my office in tears, fearing that her husband, Michael, was going to leave her because she had no desire for sex. He sat in the waiting room, looking somber.

It took more than one year to finally find the correct mix of estrogen and testosterone that suited Debra and relieved her symptoms. Now, when she comes in, her husband is seated in the waiting room with a grin on his face!

Christine, a friend of mine, was 29 when she had her uterus and ovaries removed because of endometriosis. Now 48 years old, she still has tears in her eyes when she recalls the first few years following the surgery, a time when she felt that she was not herself anymore. Her mind, her body, her hair, and her moods had all changed. Her sex drive was nonexistent. Apparently, the synthetic hormones she was receiving were not sufficient, but her health-care provider assured her that they were. Christine had no idea that she could take a larger dose of estrogen, because she considered her doctor's advice to be the final word. Many health-care providers do not realize that the younger the patient, the higher her estrogen requirements are! If the woman's ovaries are removed, she probably also needs testosterone supplementation. It was not until years later, after Christine had moved out of state, that she found a medical provider who would respond to her needs. I wish I had known her back then.

. . . **Hormone replacement therapy:** Estrogen replacement therapy may increase libido and improve other menopausal symptoms. In some cases, sexual functioning may take up to 6 to 12 months to improve.

Testosterone, given orally or transdermally, does improve sexual desire and a sense of well-being in women who have their ovaries removed. Testosterone, when added to estrogen therapy, enhances sexual activity and satisfaction among postmenopausal women even more than estrogen alone. (See chapter 5: "Hormonal Replacement Therapy").

My experience has been that when a patient complains of decreased libido, it is usually something very complex. I take some time to sort out what is going on with the patient's life as a whole, because just prescribing a pill or a cream will not necessarily make her problems go away.

When the subject of testosterone replacement was discussed on *Oprah*, there were many phone calls from women who wanted to try it. Her guest recommended that testosterone should be applied directly to the genital area to enhance a woman's sex life. For years, testosterone has been applied to the genital area among women who suffer from a condition called Lichen sclerosis et atrophicus of the vulva, which affects mostly older women, but can also be present in those who are younger. In this condition, part of the skin is thinned out and becomes irritated, with subsequent itching and thickening of some areas. If not treated, scar tissue will form, sometimes causing partial obstruction of the vaginal entrance. Long-term, topical use of testosterone or topical steroids will keep the tissue healthy. However, since it is a chronic disease, it will progress as soon as therapy is stopped.

In my opinion, testosterone does not have to be applied directly to the genital area in order to work.

. . . **Alcohol:** Alcohol removes inhibitions and may cause a woman to enter into activities that she would have morally rejected if she were not intoxicated. On the other hand, large amounts of alcohol can decrease sex drive because alcohol is a depressant.

. . . **Problems with the male partner:** An interested partner is the most important factor for good sex at any age. Women who had active sex lives in their youth are likely to do so after menopause as long as they have sexually functioning partners. Older women usually have partners who are also experiencing changes in their own sexual response and behavior. With age, a man's erectile capacity declines, or this decline may be caused by alcoholism, smoking, vascular disease, or diabetes.

Men also experience a decline in their testosterone level with age, causing a declining frequency of erection. Since men need a very small amount of testosterone, replacement therapy does not usually help. Aging also has a psychological effect on a man. He might want to have sex less frequently and may need more physical stimulation to achieve and maintain an erection. Some men may not ejaculate every time they have intercourse. A young man may have an erection within seconds of stimulation, but with advancing age, it may take several minutes before the penis becomes very firm, it becomes flaccid faster, and it takes longer to have another erection.

Older men who do not achieve erection on more than one occasion may be afraid that they are becoming impotent, causing premature ejaculation, which can make a male partner avoid sex altogether. Men can also lose their erections if they fear they will hurt a partner after gynecological surgery. Following a major illness or a heart attack, a male partner may be afraid of having sexual intercourse for fear of recurrence.[5] Some men who have problems with sexual performances may blame their partner, causing her to have psychological problems.

Many women whose partners are impotent do continue to have an active sex life. They become very creative using oral sex, manual stimulation, and sometimes a vibrator, to achieve orgasm. Some will be emotionally and physically satisfied just being able to cuddle with their partner. Some women who never enjoyed sex are grateful to let go of sex once their partner can no longer perform.

— *Male partners and impotence:* An estimated 30 million American men in their 60s, 70s, and 80s suffer from impotence, or the difficulty to obtain or maintain an erection. Impotence can be associated with illnesses such as diabetes or depression. Treatments for impotence have included injections into the penis, suppositories, implants, or vacuum devices that cause the penis to fill with blood. With Viagra, we have a phenomenon that has taken the sexual world by storm. Men used to *lie* about how often they were having sex; now they lie about being impotent just to get the prescription! The dilemma of insurance companies, which often pay for these drugs is, "What is considered to be a normal amount of sex for a man?"

When men rushed to get this miracle drug, I saw the effects in my office. Women, who for years had to repress their own sexuality because of their mate's inability to perform, were now having fulfilling sexual relationships. Others were having great difficulty coping with the renewed sense of sexual vigor on the part of their mates.

A Patient's Story

One woman whose life has been affected by Viagra is Laura, age 72, with a 77-year-old husband who had been taking the drug. They live in a trailer and have traveled all over the United States. When they came to my office, the husband did most of the talking; he requested some testosterone for his wife. I guessed that something was going on because Laura barely spoke, so I refused to have him present during the examination. Laura was relieved and started to cry. "I feel like a sex slave and a prisoner to this stranger who used to be my husband. There is no place to run or hide in the confinement of the trailer. He wants sex all the time! I am sore; I don't want it; I want out. But, I do love this man, the father of my children," she continued. "I don't know what to do." Laura was also concerned that her attitude might cause her husband to look outside their marriage for sex.

A horrifying scene came to mind . . . the Lorena Bobbitt case. (For those readers who are not familiar with it, Lorena allegedly had an abusive husband. One night she cut off his penis with a kitchen knife while he slept. Then she drove off and threw the penis in a field. This precious organ had to be retrieved and later surgically reattached.) As a concerned physician, I had to find a better alternative for Laura. So, I started her on testosterone cream, at the lowest dose, that she could apply daily to her inner thigh. It must have worked to increase her libido, because two months later I received a phone call from a contented husband requesting another refill!

❦ ❦ ❦

Communication is especially important between older couples, as they may not feel comfortable discussing sexual problems. Not being aware of sexual dysfunction that is related to aging, the subject may be taken, unfortunately, as a personal rejection. If the cause of the male dysfunction is irreversible, the couple should find alternatives to intercourse. Manual simulation and using a vibrator are options for bringing a woman to orgasm.

I would like to add that, contrary to popular belief, women haven't flocked to their gynecologists requesting Viagra for themselves! Viagra, which is covered by most insurance plans for men, brought up the subject of discrimination against women in the health-care system. According to the Alan Guttmacher Institute, women pay 68 percent more in out-of-pocket costs for medical care than men. This is partly due to the cost of contraception. Most medications related to men's health are covered by insurance companies, while most young women have to pay out of pocket for their birth-control pills. Since most insurance plans do not cover birth-control pills, the American College of Obstetricians and Gynecologists, of which I am a Fellow, is looking into reversing this trend. Just before Viagra arrived on the market, then-Governor Pete Wilson of California vetoed a bill that would require insurance to pay for birth-control pills because it did not include an exemption for religious employers who objected to the use of contraception. This undermined the effort of many obstetricians (including myself, a feminist who worked hard to have this bill passed).

. . . **Orgasm:** An orgasm is an ecstatic feeling, the result of erotic stimulation. It takes a woman an average of five to seven minutes of stimulation to reach an orgasm. The time involved depends upon the adequacy of the stimulation. The average woman reaches a climax with intercourse about 50 percent of the time, and 95 percent by masturbation.

The Graffenberg spot, or G-spot, is a very sensitive area of the vagina, located at the base of the bladder. When stimulated, a woman can easily reach an orgasm.

Antidepressants such as Zoloft, Paxil, Fluoxetine, Sertraline, and Paroxetine may delay orgasm. Some patients using these drugs have complained of anorgasmia, or inability to have orgasms.

Other patients have reported that after menopause, the intensity of their orgasm diminished. Some agree that it does improve after using testosterone.

— *Delay or absence of orgasm:* About 10 percent of women never experience an orgasm. More than 50 percent of women are unable to regularly attain orgasm during coitus. Only 30 percent of women regularly have orgasm with intercourse. Another 20 percent reach orgasm if their partners add clitoral stimulation.

Faking an orgasm is something many women do; it may be symptomatic of larger issues in the relationship. One of the main reasons women "fake it" is so they won't offend a partner. Women can fake orgasms in many situations: when they're tired, worried about family problems or about getting pregnant, disenchanted with their partner, or just to get it over with as soon as possible.

Now women confess that they fake orgasms to appease their partners who are on Viagra!

. . . **Masturbation:** The act of touching oneself, and experiencing sexual arousal leading to orgasm, is very natural. Masturbation has, unfortunately, been erroneously associated with many mental and physical diseases and even silly things such as hair growing on the palms! Many religions condemn masturbation as a sin. It is natural during infancy that, while touching their bodies, children experience pleasure; however, the child is told again and again not to do this, and is soon convinced that it is taboo. Children will continue to masturbate where adults cannot see them.

More and more people are choosing masturbation as a way to release sexual tension. In an age when everyone should be concerned about sexually transmitted disease, some couples are choosing masturbation as a way to please each other until they are sure that neither partner is infected with the HIV virus. Mutual masturbation can enhance a couple's sex life.

Many women are sexually inactive because they do not currently have a partner. In the United States today, there are only 69 men for every 100 women aged 65 and older. This gap is expected to increase, leaving more older females without companions. Older women usually outlive their partners, and as such, should know that masturbation can be a safe alternative. It can also teach a woman who is having difficulty achieving an orgasm with a partner to pleasure herself, and then she can show her partner what works best. Fantasizing is very common during masturbation and may be helpful to aid sexual arousal. A woman can enjoy sexual arousal both through masturbation and with a partner.

About 80 percent of women, and even more men, engage in self-pleasuring, either frequently or occasionally. Masturbation helps to relieve tension when a spouse is ill, or when the frequency of the partner's desire for intercourse differs. Women who achieve orgasm with masturbation are more likely to reach orgasm with a partner. To maintain a healthy vaginal mucosa, masturbation, in the absence of a sexual partner, is important.

. . . Birth control: If women are fertile, they can still become pregnant until they reach menopause. Older women have a high percentage of unintended pregnancies and subsequent abortions.[6] If you are perimenopausal and sexually active, you will need to use some type of birth control to avoid unwanted pregnancy until you have had no periods for 12 consecutive months.

For some of my perimenopausal patients who are experiencing hot flashes and other symptoms related to the decline of estrogen, I recommend a very low dose of estrogen. However, I make sure to tell them that this is not enough to prevent pregnancy.

In choosing a birth-control method, you must evaluate how it will affect your life. Will it diminish the spontaneity of lovemaking? Are you comfortable enough to insert birth-control devices before having sex? What about your partner? If the birth-control method must be used each time prior to intercourse, is it effective in preventing pregnancy? Does it also protect against sexually transmitted disease (STDs)?

Every fertile woman should keep this in mind: Except for abstinence, no birth-control method is 100 percent effective against pregnancy, HIV (the AIDS virus), or other types of STDs.

Hormone-based birth-control methods—the Pill, the skin implant Norplant, the injection Depo-Provera, and the IUD (intrauterine device)—are most effective. They're far more effective than methods that must be used each time you have intercourse, which include the male and female condom, diaphragm, spermicides, films, cervical cap, rhythm method, withdrawal, or natural family planning.

Approximately 5 percent of women who use the Pill for more than five years may notice an increase of blood pressure above 140/90 mmhg.

The methods that include the use of spermicides, especially those containing Nonoxynol-9, have a better chance of protecting against some forms of STDs. When condoms are used along with another form of birth control, the chance of avoiding both pregnancy and STDs is higher.

— *Emergency contraception, or "morning after"*: What if your birth-control method has failed, or you're not sure it was used properly? Medications and procedures are now available to prevent pregnancy by preventing maturation of the fertilized egg. If you think you may need emergency contraception, contact your health-care provider as soon as possible after the sexual activity, but preferably no later than 72 hours afterward. Or, you can call 888-NOT-2-LATE to hear information about how you can prevent pregnancy after sex.

. . . **Sexually transmitted diseases (STDs):** All sexually active, premenopausal women with male partners need protection from unwanted pregnancy, as well as protection against STDs. Postmenopausal women do not need to worry about pregnancy prevention but still need to protect themselves against STDs.

Some questions that need to be answered before engaging in intercourse with a new partner are:

- How many sexual partners did he have in the past year?
- Did he use a condom with every sexual partner?
- Do you know your partner's sexual habits?
- Has your partner had any blood transfusions?
- Has your partner had any STDs?
- Does your partner intend to be faithful?

The most common STDs in the United States are chlamydia, herpes, gonorrhea, syphilis, genital warts, trichomoniasis, hepatitis B, hepatitis C, and HIV (human immunodeficiency virus) or AIDS (Acquired Immunodeficiency Syndrome). HIV is the virus responsible for AIDS. Several other diseases occur but are less common. Granuloma inguinale and chancroid are characterized by painful genital ulcers and the formation of pus in the lymph nodes of the groin. Lymphogranuloma venereum, caused by a member of the chlamydia group of organisms, creates a sore, inflammation, and pus in the lymph system. Two insect-caused skin diseases can also be transmitted sexually—scabies (caused by mites), and pediculosis pubis (caused by lice).

According to a study financed by the National Institute of Allergy and Infectious Diseases, women are twice as likely as men to contact gonorrhea, hepatitis B, and other STDs, with minority women disproportionately affected.

Most of these diseases can be prevented by changing lifestyles, principally through abstinence or maintaining a monogamous relationship, and avoiding sexual contact with people who have genital sores or high-risk lifestyles.

— HIV/AIDS and the older woman: Older women who find themselves divorced from a high-school sweetheart may have difficulties entering the dating game, but they still need to practice safe sex. About 60,000 individuals over the age of 50 have full-blown AIDS, and about 10 percent of all new AIDS cases are individuals age 50 and older.

I recommend to my patients that, when they meet a new partner, regardless of how clean and healthy he may appear, they should not engage in intercourse until he has been tested for the HIV virus. Also, they should remember that it may take up to one year for an infected person to have a positive test. Some men may be reluctant to get tested. I tell my patients that if that man really cares for them, he should understand and cooperate.

Perimenopausal and postmenopausal women are more at risk of acquiring HIV because of the changes that occur in the vagina with aging (there is less lubrication, and the walls of the vagina become thin). The older female entering a new relationship might not feel comfortable talking about STD prevention.

HIV is no longer considered a disease of gay men. Over the years, the pattern of HIV infection has changed from primarily affecting men to affecting both genders equally. According to a recent study, HIV-infected women show lower survival rates than men. The risks of developing most AIDS-related infections were similar for women and men, although women did have an increased risk for bacterial pneumonia and a reduced risk for Kaposi's sarcoma. Women infected with HIV have a 30 percent higher risk of dying from AIDS than do men over the same time period, despite the fact that HIV progresses at the same rate in both sexes.

It can be very difficult for women to ask a partner to use a condom. In some cases, sex is used as power. It can be very hard for a woman in an abusive relationship to refuse sex with a partner, even when she is afraid of STDs and pregnancy. Among some cultures, the macho attitude exists, "You are my wife; you are mine; you have no right to tell me when I should have sex and what I should do or not do; and by the way, I can always get it somewhere else."

Women need to stop seeing themselves as victims and discover how powerful they really are.

It is important to take charge of your sexuality, enjoy sex, and protect yourself at the same time. Use condoms, and get tested!

Improving Your Sex Life

Learning techniques that involve pleasurable touching, and enhancing communication skills so you and your partner can tell each other what feels good, can be much more effective than psychotherapy.

Ways to increase interest in sex include: fantasy, music, sexy movies, books, communicating desires, and making time for sexual intimacy a high priority. Plan a vacation or a weekend together alone. A healthy lifestyle, stress control, and regular exercise can improve a depressed mood. Busy people tend to go to bed early, so make time for yourself and make time for sex! One way to make sex work for years is to "treat each other as lovers."[7]

In case of marital conflicts, both parties will benefit from seeing a marital counselor. Many of my patients who have experienced sexual difficulties have responded very well with psychotherapy.

Conclusion

Continued sexual activity is a desired and important part of a woman's life. Although there may be some complications related to aging, they should not become permanent obstacles to a woman's sexual fulfillment. Every female should become aware of age-related dysfunction and search for practical means of coping, always staying open to the idea of seeing health-care professionals with expertise in treating sexual dysfunction. No matter what their age, women can lead a sexually active and fulfilled life!

CHAPTER 18

Healthy Aging

by Louise L. Hay

There are events in life that are considered "destiny experiences." Meeting Dr. Carolle was definitely one of those times. I was attending a four-day workshop given by Dr. Andrew Weil and Dr. Christiane Northrup, and on the fourth day, during Dr. Northrup's question-and-answer period, a striking looking woman arose. She introduced herself as Dr. Carolle Jean-Murat from San Diego, and began to ask the most interesting, intelligent questions. I thought to myself, *This is a dynamite, powerful woman, and I must meet her.*

At the break, I introduced myself to her, and we had an instant soul connection. It was as though we had always known each other. I love strong women, and Dr. Carolle was powerful, beautiful, and filled with the most wonderful vitality. We agreed to meet for lunch, and the rest is history.

As the owner and publisher of Hay House, I am honored to be publishing this important book. I believe that it is vital that women are given the opportunity to explore all the many avenues of healing that are open to them. Only in this way can we learn to take charge of our own health and our own healing processes. The pharmaceutical companies want to sell us their products, so their information and advertising is very biased.

Dr. Carolle is a dedicated physician who truly cares for women and has a vast repertoire of knowledge and experience to draw upon. She is my personal gynecologist, and I am an informed patient. Together we work as a team to keep my body as healthy as possible.

A New Perspective on Aging

The ways in which we currently age have been programmed into us, and we have accepted this idea as a reality. As a society, with some exceptions, we have come to believe that we all will get old, sick, senile, frail, and die—in that order. This does not have to be the truth for us any longer.

As we refuse to accept these old fears and beliefs, this can become a time for us to begin to reverse the negative parts of the aging process. The current crop of baby boomers is not going to sit back and age like their parents did. We will live longer, and if we take charge of our health, we will live exciting, productive lives.

I believe that the second half of our lives can be even more wonderful than the first half—we can definitely make these years exciting ones. If we want to age successfully, then we must make a conscious choice to do so. Healthy aging is learning how to keep the life force strong within us. We can do this with self-love, and with good food and exercise.

Staying healthy into our later years is an act of loving ourselves. We can make deliberate choices to care for who we are. We can study books on nutrition in order to learn to fuel our bodies with the most nutritious foods possible. I don't like to talk about diet; rather, I choose to talk about food choices. We can explore some form of exercise to keep our bones strong and our bodies flexible. We can read books or listen to tapes or take classes that teach our how to use our minds. We can learn how to think in ways that support a peaceful, loving, healthy life.

Whenever I see older women who are frail, ill, and incapacitated, I know I am often looking at a lifetime of inadequate nutrition, lack of exercise, and an accumulation of years of negative thoughts and beliefs. So many of the problems we face in our later years come from the lifestyle choices we made when we were younger.

We women need to learn how to take care of our magnificent bodies so that we can sail into our older years in perfect physical shape. I had a physical recently, and the doctor told me I was in "amazingly good physical condition for someone my age." It disturbed me that he expected a woman of 72 to be in poor health.

Living a Healthful Life

Fast food and processed, packaged foods do not support life. No matter how pretty and mouth-watering the picture on the package, there is no life in these foods. Our bodies need fresh, living foods, such as fresh fruits, salads, vegetables, grains; and small amounts of meats, poultry, and fish. These are the foods that will sustain our bodies well into old age.

You may not want to hear this, but Soul Food is also "heart attack food." It may please the tastebuds, but eaten consistently over a lifetime, it contributes to all sorts of health problems.

As teenagers, we can get away with a lot of poor food choices. We may not feel our best, but at least we're not sick. However, when we reach our mid-40s, our past food history begins to catch up with us. This is when so many women find that their bodies are not working well, and the diseases start to manifest.

Don't listen to the dairy or meat industries. They don't care about your health; they're only interested in profits. Eating lots of red meat and dairy products are not good for women's bodies. Caffeine and sugar are two other culprits that contribute to many of the problems that women face with their health.

Ask yourself, "How do I want to age?" Observe women who are aging miserably, and notice those who are aging magnificently. What do these two groups do differently? Are *you* willing to do what it takes to be healthy, happy, and fulfilled in your later years?

Almost all the research done on older people has been by the pharmaceutical industry on disease and what is "wrong" with us and what drugs we require. There is a need to do in-depth studies on older women who are healthy, happy, fulfilled, and enjoying their lives. The more we study what is "right" with older women, the more we will know how we can all accomplish healthy living.

How to Accept and Love Our Bodies

It is crucial to our well-being to constantly love and appreciate ourselves. Loving our bodies is important at any stage of our lives, but it is absolutely vital as we grow older. Anger is not healing. If we put anger into any part of our bodies, especially a part that is sick, it only delays the healing process. If there is some part of your body that you are not happy with, then take a month or so and put love into that area on a daily basis. Tell your body that you love it: "I love you, body! I really, really love you."

What if part of your body is sagging or wrinkled? This part has been with you for a lifetime, and it is doing the best it can with the health choices you have made. Hating your body will not make it young and beautiful. Love your body, and it will love you back. Your hips and breasts and your face and your skin will be with you for the rest of your life. Take care of your body, and love every bit of it—from the top of your head down to the tips of your toes—and all the organs in between. When you love yourself, others love you, too, and you will be irresistibly attractive all your life.

I am a great believer in the philosophy that our thoughts and our words shape our experiences. So we can quite unknowingly, just by thinking, contribute to our health or to our diseases. Dr. Candace Pert discovered "neuropeptides." These are the chemical messengers in our brain that travel to every part of our body, touching every cell and depositing a bit of that chemical in it. They do this each time we think a thought or speak a word.

If our thoughts are fearful, angry, or in any way negative, then the chemicals these messengers deposit "depress" our immune systems. If our thoughts are loving, optimistic, and positive, then the different chemicals these messengers, or neuropeptides, deposit will "enhance" our immune systems.

So, moment by moment, we are consciously or unconsciously choosing healthy thoughts or unhealthy thoughts. Poisonous thoughts poison our bodies. We cannot allow ourselves to indulge in negative thinking. It is making us sick and killing us.

In addition to making sound choices for ourselves nutritionally and medically, we need to take charge of our thinking. Negative thinking produces negative experiences. If we want to change our lives for the better, we must learn to think thoughts that support us and help improve the quality of our lives. When we love and appreciate who we are, we naturally take better care of ourselves.

My Personal Health Routines

I am entering my 73rd year, and I am extremely healthy. I eat lots of organic fresh fruits, vegetables, and grains, along with some fish and chicken. Once a week I go on a fresh juice fast. Twice a year I go to the Optimum Health Institute in Lemon Grove, California, and do a week or two on their raw foods cleansing program. It does absolute wonders for cleaning my body and clearing my mind. I have so much energy when I leave there, and my thinking is sharp and clear.

I exercise several times a week using the Pilates method, I work out in the gym with machines and weights, and I have just recently taken up kick boxing. Kick boxing is strenuous, and I may not stay with it forever, but it is lots of fun for now, and I love doing new things. Weather permitting, I swim. My dog always wants to take a walk, so I keep active and my body loves it.

First thing in the morning, I do a little "mirror work." I look into my eyes in the mirror and say, "You are wonderful, and I love you. What can I do today to make you happy?" This simple mirror work has done such wonders for me. There was a time when I could hardly look into my own eyes. Now I just adore myself. Please join me in this life-changing exercise. Even if it feels foolish, keep it up. At night, say, "I love you. Now sleep well, and I will see you in the morning."

I also meditate each morning—that is to say, I sit quietly and give myself time to connect with the inner wisdom that is within all of us. I express gratitude for all the good I have in my life. I affirm that I deserve to have a great day and that I am open and receptive to only good experiences. I declare that my health is excellent, and I send love to every part of my life.

If a problem comes up during the day, I stop and say to myself, *"All is well. Everything is working out for my highest good. Out of this situation, only good will come."* This statement keeps me from getting into negative thinking.

In the evening before I go to sleep, I express gratitude for everything that happened that day, including any lessons or challenges that came my way. I bless my body with love, and thank it for being with me for another day. Then I bless all my experiences with love and drift off to sleep peacefully.

🦋 🦋 🦋

Just because the years are passing does not mean that the quality of our lives must automatically go downhill. Menopause is a time for women's wisdom to come forth in new and different ways. As we tap into this wisdom, new possibilities open for us. It is never too late for us to dream and to have goals. We will have so much more time left these days, so let's see how we can live it to the fullest. What can we do and explore and experience that our mothers and our grandmothers had no chance to do?

Think about what you would really love to do with the next portion of your life. Don't think of limitations or why you can't do things. Allow your mind to go in new directions. You have a lifetime ahead of you, so fill it with experiences that will fulfill you. When you are clear in your mind about what you really want and know that you deserve to have it, then the Universe will find avenues for this to come to you—probably in ways you would not expect.

So stay healthy and enjoy your life. There is so much to see and do and experience!

Self-Talk for the Mind and Body

I would like to leave you with some powerful affirmations that you can say on a daily basis to improve your health and the quality of your life.

I LOVE MY BODY—EVERY PART OF IT—INSIDE AND OUT.

I LOVE MY FACE.

I LOVE MY BREASTS.

I LOVE MY STOMACH.

I LOVE MY GENITALS.

I LOVE MY THIGHS.

I AM AT PEACE WITH MENOPAUSE.

I HAVE HEALING POWERS.

ALL IS WELL IN MY BODY.

I AM FAR MORE THAN ANY DIS-EASE; I AM THE SOLUTION.

I AM SAFE, AND ALL IS WELL.

I LIVE IN PEACE AND HARMONY.

ALL IS WELL IN MY RELATIONSHIPS.

I AM DESIRABLE.

I AM A SEXY, SENSUAL WOMAN.

I LOVE AND ACCEPT EVERYTHING ABOUT MYSELF.

I AM SAFE, AND THE UNIVERSE LOVES ME.

CHAPTER 19

Take Charge of Your
Overall Health

Visit Your Health-Care Provider Regularly

As a doctor, I know that a visit to a health-care provider isn't at the top of your list of good times, especially when it comes to the pelvic exam (which includes a look at your vaginal interior). Most women dread the experience! But a physical exam is one of the vital steps for maintaining good health. A woman should have an annual physical exam, including a Pap smear if she is 18 or older, or at any age if she is sexually active.

I am not sure which I hate most—going to the gynecologist or going to the dentist. Although I'm a gynecologist myself, when I am on that table, underneath that paper gown, I am a patient like everyone else. The actress Cher, while playing a gynecologist in a movie, said, "You are never too rich, never too young, and never too far from the end of the table."

Repeatedly, my patients ask, "By the way, Doc, do you do your own Pap smears?" We usually have a good laugh when I try to demonstrate the acrobatics that would be required to accomplish that feat. Then I say, "The doctor who treats herself has a fool for a patient."

Choosing the right doctor can be a very sensitive affair. After all, a gynecologist is someone who, after a few minutes of talk, is going to see you completely undressed and then poke around the most intimate parts of your body. Most patients choose a gynecologist they like and stay with him or her for life, whether they are covered by an insurance plan or not.

In most industrialized countries where women are concerned about prevention and can afford it, it is routine for them to visit their gynecologist for annual examinations. In other parts of the world, or among some transplanted cultures in America, it is not common at all. In some countries, an unmarried woman cannot have a Pap smear or breast exam regardless of her age. To do so would be an admission that she is a sexual being, which is completely taboo. Because she is unmarried, the idea of sexual activity is not only immodest, but repugnant to her culture. Any pelvic exam where a foreign object, including fingers, is inserted into the vagina or disrupts the hymen, is not acceptable.

In other cultures, visiting a gynecologist can risk destroying proof of virginity. It is often very important for a woman to be a virgin before marriage. In some societies, the bloodstained sheet, proving consummation of the marriage, is hung out the window by the groom's family for the town to inspect. Without the bloodstain, some brides meet an "accidental" death.

A Personal Story

Just like every other patient, I have to work up the courage to call for an appointment with my gynecologist. There have been times when I've been able to delay this dreaded encounter for weeks at a time. First, I've had to cancel because of an emergency. Then I had a yeast infection followed by my period. Then my gynecologist had to cancel because of a delivery. But eventually the reality of the visit had to be faced.

It starts the night before. That's when I look at the calendar and realize, "Tomorrow is THE day." I usually refrain from intercourse, which is what I recommend to my own patients. I also advise against douching.

When I wake up in the morning and realize what is going to happen, the discomfort sets in. What am I going to wear? Where is my best underwear? What about my shoes? My feet sweat, and my shoes don't always smell so great, so I choose new shoes, or shoes that have been waiting for months at the back of my closet for a special occasion. I have to wear a brand new pair of pantyhose. While I'm getting dressed, I look at the crop of hair in my armpits. Should I shave? I grew up in a culture where shaving was not part of a woman's body ritual. Will I feel self-conscious if I don't? What about my toenails? Are they clean enough? They're going to be hanging out on either side of the doctor's face. By the time I'm in the car, I'm hoping that I'll be paged on an emergency call so I can delay the inevitable again. And I can't even think about the possibility that something might turn up in the exam, even though I'm aware of all the things that can go wrong.

When I finally arrive, I remind the nurse taking my blood pressure and weight that I hate the whole thing. "Do you have to weigh me? I'm sure that I have regained all of the pounds I lost last year." "Yes, I do," she tells me sweetly. My gynecologist, Myelin Ho, knows that I hate to sit dressed in those embarrassing paper gowns, so she rarely makes me wait. "There you are, finally," she will tell me with her warm smile. "Let's do it and get over with it." I grunt.

While I'm stretched out on the hard, cold examining table, she tries to talk to me while her gentle hands are examining my body. Looking up, I laugh as I remember that in one office I'd had, I placed signs on the ceiling to be read while patients were lying on the table. One said, "Don't worry, nobody is perfect, except you." Another one said, "Patience is a virtue, even in a situation like this." And the last one, my patients' favorite, is, "Stop complaining, I have to go through it, too!"

I feel tense. "Go limp," I keep repeating to myself, while I am trying to disappear from the face of the earth. "It's over," she finally says. "Everything is in perfect condition." "Thank God," I say to myself. As soon as she leaves the room, I jump off the table, get dressed, and run away.

As Grandma used to say, "Everything does come to an end."

❦ ❦ ❦

It's important to choose a health-care provider who makes you feel comfortable, doesn't hurry during the exam, is sympathetic to your doubts and fears, listens carefully to you, and welcomes and answers all your questions.

— **Annual health checkups:** An annual physical exam is an excellent way to detect most health problems early rather than late. Your health-care provider will perform tests appropriate to your age. During each visit, your weight and blood pressure will be recorded. If you're over 40, a urine sample will be taken. This is also a good opportunity for your health-care provider to review your medical history and that of your family. Knowing your family's health status helps your health-care provider diagnose, prevent, and treat diseases. Routine tests performed during your visit can uncover problems even before symptoms are present.

Prevent Disease—It's the Best Medicine

When an illness is diagnosed early, treatment has the greatest potential for resulting in a cure. The majority of diseases, including cancer, can be successfully treated if they're discovered early. That is why prevention and early detection is preferable.

Good health is related to self-esteem. Black women are more likely to suffer from prejudice and racism, which erodes their self-esteem and affects their health. Black women are less likely than white women to practice preventive health; subsequently, they tend to be diagnosed when a disease is already in an advanced stage, with less possibility of cure. Ethnic minority women, including blacks, are more likely to be poor, not as well educated, and have less access to health-care education than white women.

White women and women of higher economic status are more likely to be treated effectively than other women.[1] There is a need for reforms in public policies and health-care systems and intervention programs, as well as effective intervention at the societal and individual level, which will benefit ethnic minority women.

Consult a health-care provider in case of a nagging cough, persistent hoarse voice, problems with swallowing, unusual bleeding or discharge, any unusual lump or discharge from the breast, or a sore that does not heal. Home remedies can help with some mild forms of illness. However, serious illness such as cancer calls for a specialist and hospital treatment. Be sure to pay attention to symptoms that do not go away, and take the steps to put yourself in competent hands.

Colorectal Cancer

Colorectal cancer, or cancer of the colon and rectum, is the third leading cause of cancer death for women, behind lung and breast cancers, most often striking those over the age of 50. According to a report in the *Journal of Women's Health*, only 10 to 20 percent of women over age 50 are tested for colon cancer, mainly because they believe that this cancer strikes more men than women. Colorectal cancer is expected to strike 67,000 women in 1999, compared to 62,400 men. An estimated 28,800 women and 27,800 men are expected to die from it.

Colorectal cancer screening: Like all cancers, the earlier colorectal cancer is detected, the more effective the treatment will be. You should have a digital ("by finger") rectal exam after the age of 50 to check the stool for signs of blood (fecal hemocult). Your health-care provider may ask you to take a stool sample at home and place it on a special card and return it to the office to be tested.

Another screening test for colorectal cancer is sigmoidoscopy. Sigmoidoscopy is the visualization of the rectum and the lower portion of the colon. During the exam, the walls of the colon are examined and a sample of tissues (biopsy) can be taken if anything unusual is noted. For women at low risk of developing colorectal cancer, sigmoidoscopy can be started at age 50, and repeated every three to five years.

For women over age 40 who have a history of inflammatory bowel disease such as ulcerative colitis and Crohn's disease, polyps in the colon, or a family history of colon cancer, a colonoscopy—not a sigmoidoscopy—should be performed. During colonoscopy, the rectum and the full length of the colon are examined. An alternative would be to have a sigmoidoscopy plus a barium enema.

PATIENTS' STORIES

Recently, I received a large bouquet of lovely sweet-pea flowers from a patient named Lois, who had no children. About 11 years ago, during her annual exam, her fecal hemocult was positive. Her colonoscopy revealed a small cancer, which was surgically removed. Lois did not like the idea of staying in the hospital. Walking through the hospital gift shop, I saw a cute little bear that looked just like her, and bought it for her. I knew that it would put a smile on her face. Since then, every year, I get a gift from Lois. When I tell her that she does not need to do this, she says, "You saved my life. I want to do it, so let me."

Helen, a 71-year-old patient, came to my office two years ago. She was very proud of herself because, she told me, she'd had her mammogram the day before. In addition, she had seen her cardiologist who checked her lipid profile, which was normal. She had been watching her diet, was exercising regularly, and was scheduled for a sigmoidoscopy with her internist the following week. I recalled that, during the previous year, Helen's younger sister had been diagnosed with a colon cancer that was discovered very high in the colon. "You need more than a sigmoidoscopy," I told her. "You have to have a colonoscopy." She went back to her internist and insisted that she be referred to a gastroenterologist, who scheduled the colonoscopy. A small cancer was detected high in the colon, and a simple resection of the area, by a general surgeon, cured her. A sigmoidoscopy would have missed it.

❦ ❦ ❦

If you have a family history of colon cancer, you should start having a colonoscopy ten years before the age at which your youngest relative was diagnosed with the cancer. If you observe any change in bowel movements, or any rectal bleeding or blood in the stool, you should consult your health-care provider.

Pap Smears

Cancer of the cervix is a good example of how prevention and early detection make life better. Cervical cancer is the most frequent deadly cancer in developing countries where prevention is lacking. The Pap test to screen for cervical cancer was introduced in 1950 and soon became widely used in the United States. The result? With early detection and treatment, the number of deaths from cervical cancer dropped from 8,487 in 1960, to 4,800 in 1996, while the size of the sexually active female population increased considerably.

Vision Screening

Glaucoma—damage to the optic nerve caused by elevated pressure within the eye—is the leading cause of preventable blindness. Glaucoma is present in 5 percent of the population age 40 and above. Blacks have a significantly higher risk of developing glaucoma than people of other races. People with diabetes are three times more likely to develop glaucoma.

Loss of vision due to glaucoma is permanent and irreversible, so it is very important to discover glaucoma early and treat it adequately. A quick, simple, and painless test can easily diagnose the presence or absence of glaucoma. Starting at age 40, you should have this test performed by an optometrist, a family physician, or an ophthalmologist.

Skin Cancer

More than 500,000 Americans develop skin cancer each year, and the number is rising. Over 90 percent of skin cancer occurs on skin that is exposed to ultraviolet light. Everyone is at risk for skin cancer, even people with naturally dark skin. About 2,700 women die each year from melanoma, the most serious form of skin cancer.

You should avoid too much exposure to the sun, especially midday sun. Wear clothing that covers most parts of the body, and use an SPF 15 sunblock to protect exposed skin. Watch out for moles that are larger than a pencil eraser, have variations in color, and those that have irregular borders. Any unusual skin lesions, or changes in a birthmark or mole, should be checked by a physician.

For further help, use the UV (ultraviolet) Index. This index translates the day's amount of cancer-related UV radiation into safe tanning minutes for your skin type. This information is indicated on the label of sunscreen products and cosmetics.

Injury Prevention

There were 42,000 people who died on United States roads in 1997 (compared to approximately 46,000 deaths from breast cancer). Sixty-three percent of those who died in car crashes were not belted at the time.

The simple act of wearing a seat belt while driving can avoid grave injuries in case of an accident. It is now required by law in many states.

Domestic Violence

Many public health experts consider violence to be an epidemic. Domestic violence is a part of this epidemic in America. About 1.8 million women are abused by their spouses each year—beatings, emotional humiliation, and rape are some examples.

From genital mutilation in African nations, forced child prostitution in Asia, dowry killings in India, and domestic violence in the United States, millions of women from every class in every country live under the threat of abuse. This can debilitate a women physically, psychologically, and socially, affecting the social health and economic development of all societies. Abused women are more susceptible to increased health problems compared to women who are not abused.[2] Between 6 to 30 percent of emergency room visits by women are due to symptoms related to abuse.[3]

In the United States, the law grants women and men equal status, making such "traditional" atrocities as being stoned to death for infidelity unheard of in this country. Still, older social and religious codes, which give informal approval for men to control "their" women, are widely practiced. Such practices occur in all walks of life, from the richest to the poorest, regardless of education, and from all ethnic and religious backgrounds. Even in the United States, it's estimated that 16 percent of women—one out of six—are victimized by violence perpetrated by their mates.

Sometimes a woman feels she is partly to blame for domestic abuse, is afraid to be stigmatized, is unwilling to break up the family, and continues to love her partner in spite of the abuse. The way to end the violence would be to leave. But, women often stay because of physical, financial, and psychological dependency and fear for themselves and their children. They can be isolated, unable to afford child care, and therefore, unable to work. Because their children are also being abused, they are afraid to leave them behind. Finally, battering may change a woman psychologically, making her believe that the abuse is her own fault since she's "not a good" wife or mother.

The situation is improving slowly. Rape—once considered an inevitable by-product of male behavior during wartime—has been declared a war crime by the United Nations. And multiple articles about domestic violence in medical literature, plus increased media coverage, are raising the awareness of health-care providers.

In addition, the idea that any type of forced sex—by a date or other friend—is rape, is gradually being accepted by men as well as women. Still, progress is slow. According to a recent report by the United States Senate Majority staff, more women than ever before are living in fear, with more than 70,000 women being sexually assaulted each year. Only one out of five rapes was committed by someone unknown to the victim—and it's estimated that only 7 percent of rapes are reported to authorities. Victims are still blamed for the crime.

If you find yourself in this situation, you can take control! You may feel humiliated, isolated, and afraid to be examined medically, but you are not alone. Counseling and support groups (low-cost or free) are available in most communities to help you find strength, so realize that you are not to blame and bring the perpetrator into the criminal justice system.

Help is just a phone call away. Just pick up the phone and call the National Council on Child Abuse and Family Violence from anywhere in the United States: (800) 222-2000.

A Personal Story

Grandma always told me that abuse should never be tolerated. She illustrated this with a story about her and my grandfather, Emmanuel. She was the mother of two small children, and the wife of a man who refused to work because of alcohol addiction and political problems. He was physically abusive to his son, my father, whenever he was home. Life was hard; Grandma took in seamstress work to pay the rent and care for the children. One day, following a small argument, my grandfather slapped Grandma on the face. She decided to make sure that he never hit her again. While he was dozing on the porch, she grabbed a hot pressing iron and hit him with it. "Don't you ever hit me again," she told him, calmly handing him ice. "This will keep it from swelling. The next time you hit me, I will cut your hand off." He never hit her again.

The drunkenness and verbal abuse continued. When she decided that she could not take it anymore, she packed his clothes and told him to leave. This was a brave move, since the church and society believed that a woman was the property of her husband. She supported the household with her hard work, and took the vows of celibacy. She was only 30 years old.

❧ ❧ ❧

Abuse does not have to be physical; it can also be mental, and both are just as scarring, hurtful, and humiliating. When a woman remains in an abusive relationship, she too can become abusive to those around her.

Table 19-a
YOUR ROUTINE CHECKUP LIST

Test/Immunization	How Often
Fecal occult blood	Yearly, beginning at age 50
Influenza vaccine	Yearly, beginning at age 55
Lipid profile (cholesterol)	Every five years beginning at age 20 and more frequently if abnormal
Mammography	Every one to two years from age 40, yearly beginning at age 50
Pap test	You and your health-care provider should decide
Sigmoidoscopy/ colonoscopy	Every three to five years after age 50
Tetanus-diphtheria booster	Every 10 years

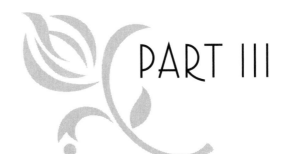

PART III

For
Further
Reference

CHAPTER 20

Making the Right Decisions

Hormonal replacement therapy (HRT) is being touted as the way to decrease a woman's risk of cardiovascular disease, osteoporosis, colon cancer, and Alzheimer's disease, among other conditions—a way to help a woman stay young and healthy, improve her quality of life, and extend her life expectancy. But every woman ages differently, depending on her health, heredity, and personality. Not everyone is a candidate for HRT.

The individualized approach toward menopause management is more challenging than ever. Estrogen replacement therapy (ERT) is contraindicated for some women, while others opt not to take estrogen. Some women cannot tolerate the side effects of HRT, and some are concerned about the potential increased risk for breast cancer.

It is true that HRT can offer the above benefits, but it may not be appropriate to use it as a first line of defense. There should be a differentiation between risk factors that one cannot modify, such as body type and heredity, and those that are modifiable, such as diet and lifestyle. Risk factors that can be modified with lifestyle choices include proper nutrition (foods low in saturated fat and rich in fiber, antioxidant, and fish oil); regular exercise; stress reduction; relaxation; and maintaining a normal body weight.

Disease risk and prevention is very complex and includes the following factors: genetics, socioeconomic situation, culture, and racial differences. A woman cannot hope to make an informed decision until a complete evaluation of her personal risk profile for heart disease, osteoporosis, and breast cancer has been done.

The Concept of Risk and What It Means to You

A risk factor describes a physical characteristic or a specific practice that increases the likelihood of disease. For example, prolonged immobilization is a risk for osteoporosis. A small increase in risk for a disease that you are already at increased risk to develop is more important than a large increase for a disease that you are unlikely to get. You should be very concerned about taking HRT for more than five years if you have a strong family history of breast cancer, because prolonged use of HRT has been linked to an increased risk of this type of cancer. On the other hand, you may not be concerned about developing breast cancer if you have an increased risk for developing heart disease, but no risk or low risk for developing breast cancer.

My Personal Point of View

Until recently, when a postmenopausal woman came to see me, I would prescribe HRT if there were no contraindications, and I might even prescribe it for an indefinite period based on information available to physicians at the time. But I have since discovered that some studies I read may have been paid for by pharmaceutical companies with a vested interest in sales!

Once I began to critically review the studies, I found that many of them were observational and were incorrectly making definitive statements about heart disease risk. Definite answers will not be available until the year 2005, depending upon the results of the Women's Health Initiative Study.

I continue to research and evaluate alternative treatments for menopausal symptoms, and the value of lifestyle changes such as diet, exercise, drinking in moderation, stress reduction, smoking cessation, the use of herbs and supplements, as well as other alternative modalities. (Please check my website at **www.drcarolle.com** for updated information and research results.)

My personal opinion is that ERT or HRT should not be prescribed indiscriminately. Replacement therapy should be reserved for a woman who becomes convinced that it is right for her. She may have arrived at this decision alone, or she may have been influenced by her mother, her health-care provider, or by other sources of risk assessment, such as this very book. "Knowledge is power," and my intention is to empower women with the right information to make informed choices.

Currently, when a patient and I are discussing HRT, I make sure that she understands all the risks. I remind her that her decision is not written in stone: Each year, during her annual checkup, we will review any new personal and family information, any new products that have become available on the market, and then decide together whether she should continue HRT or not.

Is HRT the Right Choice for You?

You need to ask yourself these important questions:

Yes No

__ __ Am I at risk for disease that can be aggravated by HRT?

__ __ Do I dislike the idea of taking medication every day?

__ __ Do I believe that taking hormones for any length of time will cause breast cancer?

__ __ Do I dislike the idea of having periods again?

__ __ Do I feel that vitamins, lifestyle change, and alternative treatments are safer than HRT?

__ __ Do I believe that menopause is not a disease and that I do not need to take a drug to deal with it?

__ __ Am I favorably influenced by my mother's example, if she did well without taking hormones?

__ __ Do I dislike the idea of taking a medication for years?

The more questions you answered with a yes, the more psychological-ly unsuited you are to HRT. In that case, use this book, and the counsel of an appropriate health-care provider, to establish a health-maintenance pro-gram instead of drug therapy.

Short-term HRT (less than five years): The decision to begin HRT should depend upon how severe your symptoms are. Some women want to start HRT right away, while others want to try alternative treatments first. Remember that the choice is always yours. If you choose HRT, you should opt for the lowest possible dose that effectively alleviates your symptoms and causes the fewest side effects. Symptoms should abate within two to three weeks.

Long-term HRT (five years or more): The reason to opt for long-term HRT is primarily the prevention of heart disease and osteoporosis. This pre-vention measure requires more than five years of HRT, a period of time that has been linked with a possible increased risk of breast cancer.

Decisions about long-term estrogen therapy need to be made on an indi-vidual basis, taking into consideration a woman's personal risk of heart dis-ease, breast cancer, and osteoporosis. Caution should be taken to balance benefits and risks. If you are at high risk for heart disease, or if you have heart disease and have been on HRT for over five years, the long-term ben-efits of HRT definitely outweigh any possible risk of breast, or any other, cancer.

There is some scientific evidence that long-term estrogen use may decrease the risk of colon cancer and Alzheimer's disease. Lifestyle changes and surveillance tests such as fecal hemocult, sigmoidoscopy, and colonoscopy can greatly reduce your risk of colon cancer. The actual inci-dence of Alzheimer's disease is low in the general population. Studies avail-able to date have concluded that HRT may decrease the incidence or sever-ity of Alzheimer's disease, but more studies are needed. I cannot, in good faith, recommend long-term HRT for prevention of colon cancer and Alzheimer's to a woman who has no other risk factors.

Other cancers that are of concern for women are ovarian, uterine, and cervical cancer. Cervical cancer is not at all related to HRT. Uterine cancer is a possibility only when estrogen is not used in conjunction with a prog-estin or progesterone. There may be an increased risk associated with ovar-ian cancer and HRT.

So, how am I going to make menopause decisions easier for you? How can I help you plow through all the medical findings, your personal risk factors, and your own needs and preferences to determine whether you should take long-term HRT or not? Carefully, but *easily,* using the following easy-to-use recommendations.

Let's get started. When we're done, you'll know exactly how to deal with these issues for the rest of your life.

Assessing Your Risk for Heart Disease, Osteoporosis, and Breast Cancer

Let's assess your risk for heart disease, osteoporosis, and breast cancer. Remember that the term "at risk" does not mean you *will* contract the disease, only that your chances are greater. Using the following questionnaires as guidelines, the goal is to help you see more clearly where you stand and in what direction you should proceed. Please consult with your health-care provider before making any final decisions.

QUESTIONNAIRE I—Heart Disease
Circle any numbers that apply to you.

1. You have a sedentary lifestyle.
2. You are overweight.
3. You are under a lot of stress.
4. You have high cholesterol
5. Your HDL is less than 35.
6. You smoke.
7. You have diabetes.
8. You have high blood pressure.
9. You have a family history of heart disease (a father, brother, grandfather, or uncle who had the disease before age 55; a mother, sister, grandmother, or aunt before age 65).
10. You have findings suggestive of heart disease on your electro-cardiogram (EKG).

Questionnaire Results for Heart Disease

(−) **No risk:** None circled.

(+) **At risk:** If you have circled any of the above. You need to determine what **LEVEL** of risk you have by answering the following.

Circle each condition below that applies to you, and enter the points to the right. Add the points; the total will determine your RISK LEVEL for heart disease.

1. You have a sedentary lifestyle. **(2)** ___
2. You are overweight. **(2)** ___
3. You are under a lot of stress. **(1)** ___
4. You have high cholesterol. **(2)** ___
5. Your HDL is less than 35. **(2)** ___
6. You smoke. **(2)** ___
7. You have diabetes. **(3)** ___
8. You have high blood pressure. **(3)** ___
9. You have a family history of heart disease. **(3)** ___
10. You have findings suggestive of heart disease on your electrocardiogram (EKG). **(5)** ___

Total Points: _____

Risk Level for Heart Disease
> 0–2 points = Average Risk
> 3–4 points = Moderate Risk
> 5 or more points = High Risk

My risk level for heart disease: _____ (average, moderate, or high)

❧ ❧ ❧

QUESTIONNAIRE II—Osteoporosis

Answer **Questionnaire II-A** if your ancestors came from Europe, especially Northern Europe or Asia, or if you are a Hispanic or Native American woman. Answer **Questionnaire II-B** if you are a black woman.

Questionnaire II-A (non-black women)
Circle any numbers that apply to you.

1. You have been postmenopausal for over five years and you are not on HRT.
2. You are thin, tall, and have a low fat mass (weigh less than 127 pounds).
3. You have a family history of osteoporosis.
4. You have a history of prolonged use of steroids, anticonvulsive medications, heparin, or thyroid hormone intake.
5. You smoke.
6. You drink moderate or heavy amounts of alcohol (more than seven drinks per week).
7. You have a sedentary lifestyle.
8. You have had a bone density (BMD) test suggesting osteopenia or osteoporosis.
9. You have a history of breakage of a bone; and either complete or incomplete breakage of the hip, vertebra, and/or distal forearm after age 40.
10. You have a maternal or paternal history of hip, wrist, or spine fractures after age 50.
11. You have a history of prolonged premenopausal amenorrhea greater than a year.
12. You have a lifelong history of low calcium intake.

Questionnaire II-A Results for Osteoporosis (non-black women)
(-) **No risk**: None circled.
(+) **At risk**: If you have circled any of the above.

❧ ❧ ❧

Questionnaire II-B (black women)

Circle any numbers that apply to you.

1. You are over 60 years old and you have never been on HRT.
2. You have a family history of osteoporosis.
3. You have a history of prolonged use of steroids, anticonvulsive medications, heparin, or thyroid hormone intake.
4. You have a bone density (BMD) test suggesting osteopenia or osteoporosis.
5. You smoke.
6. You drink moderate or heavy amounts of alcohol (more than seven drinks per week).
7. You have a history of breakage of a bone; and either complete or incomplete breakage of the hip, vertebra, and/or distal forearm after age 40.
8. You have a maternal or paternal history of hip, wrist, or spine fractures after age 50.
9. You have a history of prolonged premenopausal amenorrhea greater than a year.
10. You have a lifelong history of low calcium intake.

Questionnaire II-B Results for Osteoporosis (black women)
(-) **No risk**: None circled.
(+) **At risk**: If you have circled any of the above.

If you are at risk for osteoporosis, in order to proceed, **you need to know your BMD test result**, or have an established diagnosis of osteoporosis by your health-care provider.

BMD Test Result will be either normal, or show osteopenia or osteoporosis.

My BMD Test Result = _____ (normal, osteopenia, or osteoporosis.)

❧ ❧ ❧

QUESTIONNAIRE III—Breast Cancer
Circle any numbers that apply to you.

1. You started your period early (before age 10).
2. You entered menopause late (over the age of 55).
3. You are obese.
4. You have had breast biopsies for benign disease.
5. You drink moderate or heavy amounts of alcohol (more than seven drinks/week).
6. You have not given birth to a child, or you became a mother for the first time after the age of 30.
7. Your mother, sister, half-sister, or daughter has had breast cancer.

Questionnaire III Results for Breast Cancer
(-) No risk: None circled.

(+) At risk: If you have circled any of the above. You need to determine what **LEVEL** of risk you have by answering the following. Circle each condition below that applies to you, and enter the points to the right. Add the points. The total will determine your RISK LEVEL for breast cancer.

1. You started your period early (before age 10). **(2)** ___
2. You entered menopause late (over the age of 55). **(2)** ___
3. You are obese. **(2)** ___
4. You have had breast biopsy(s) for benign disease. **(2)** ___
5. You drink moderate or heavy amounts of alcohol (more than seven drinks/week). **(2)** ___
6. You have not given birth to a child, or you became a mother for the first time after the age of 30. **(3)** ___
7. Your mother, sister, half-sister, or daughter has had breast cancer. **(5)** ___

Total Points: _____

Risk Level for Breast Cancer
0–2 points = Average Risk
3–4 points = Moderate Risk
5 or more points = High Risk

My risk level for breast cancer: _____ (average, moderate, or high)

❦ ❦ ❦

Enter your final results for Heart Disease and Breast Cancer:

If you are not at risk write in: (-)
If you are at risk write in: (+) and your level of risk: (average, moderate, or high)

       Heart Disease: (_____)
       Breast Cancer: (_____)

Putting Your Results Together

Follow directions under the Risk Group that applies to you. You will also be given options regarding your osteoporosis risk. Remember to redo the questionnaires whenever you or a first-degree relative experiences a major health change.

Please note that references are made regarding "Lifestyle Changes," "Reducing Your Risk of Cardiovascular Disease," "Bone Health," and "Breast Health." You will find them under the section: "Risk Reduction Recommendations" at the end of this chapter.

Possible Outcomes

Risk Group A (page 235)
(-) Heart Disease
(-) Breast Cancer

Risk Group B (page 236)
(+) Heart Disease
(-) Breast Cancer

Risk Group C (page 240)

(-) Heart Disease

(+) Breast Cancer

Risk Group D (page 243)

(+) Heart Disease

(+) Breast Cancer

Risk Group A:

You Have *No Risk* for heart disease or breast cancer.

(-) Heart Disease

(-) Breast Cancer

- You are currently not at risk for heart disease. Following the "Healthy Lifestyle Changes" suggestions will help you prevent future development of heart risk. You are currently not at risk for breast cancer; however, just the fact that you are getting older increases your risk. In order to maintain your present status, please follow the "Breast Health" recommendations so you will have a better chance of avoiding this deadly disease. Whether or not you want to take HRT is a personal decision.

- If you are not at risk for osteoporosis, or if you are at risk and your BMD is normal, follow the "Bone Health" suggestions to help you continue to have strong bones and prevent hip fractures in the future. You should then repeat your BMD every two to three years.

- If you are at risk for osteoporosis, and your BMD indicates osteopenia, following the "Bone Health" suggestions may be sufficient. Another option is HRT. If you are already on HRT, you may want to consider adding an androgen to your regimen, or using the proper dosage of natural progesterone. Fosamax 5 mg, or Raloxifene 60 mg are also good options. You should then repeat your BMD every two to three years.

- If you are at risk for osteoporosis and your BMD indicates osteoporosis, following the "Bone Health" suggestions may be sufficient. You can also add any of the following: HRT, HRT plus an androgen, Fosamax 10 mg, or Calcitonin. Talk to your health-care provider about obtaining bone marker levels before treatment. By repeating the levels in three to six months, you can determine if the treatment is working. You should then repeat your BMD in one to two years.

Please check my website at **www.drcarolle.com** for updated information and research results.

Remember to redo the questionnaires whenever you or a first-degree relative experiences a major health change.

Risk Group B:
You are at risk for heart disease only.

Making a Decision about Long-Term HRT
According to Your Personal Risk Level

Below are three scenarios, *only one* of which will match your personal results. Once you find the scenario that matches your results, follow the recommendations, in partnership with your personal health-care provider. Remember, the suggestions given here are only *guidelines* to help you make better decisions for the rest of your life.

SCENARIO #1

(+) Heart Disease (average)
(-) Breast Cancer

- You can reduce your risk of heart disease by following the suggestions in "Reducing Heart Disease Risks." These suggestions may be sufficient. You are currently not at risk for breast cancer; however, just the fact that you are getting older increases your risk. In order to maintain your present status, please follow the

"Breast Health" recommendations so you will have a better chance of avoiding this deadly disease. Whether or not you want to take HRT is a personal decision.

- If you are not at risk for osteoporosis, or if you are at risk and your BMD is normal, follow the "Bone Health" suggestions to help you continue to have strong bones and prevent hip fractures in the future. You should then repeat your BMD every two to three years.

- If you are at risk for osteoporosis and your BMD indicates osteopenia, following the "Bone Health" suggestions may be sufficient. If you are already on HRT, you may want to consider adding an androgen to your regimen, or using the proper dosage of natural progesterone. Fosamax 5 mg, or Raloxifene 60 mg, are also good options. You should then repeat your BMD every two to three years.

- If you are at risk for osteoporosis and your BMD indicates osteoporosis, following the "Bone Health" suggestions may be sufficient. If you are already on HRT, consider adding an androgen. Another option is Fosamax 10 mg, or Calcitonin. Talk with your health-care provider about obtaining bone marker levels before treatment. By repeating the levels in three to six months, you can determine if the treatment is working. You should then repeat your BMD in one to two years.

Please check my website at **www.drcarolle.com** for updated information and research results.

Remember to redo the questionnaires whenever you or a first-degree relative experiences a major health change.

SCENARIO # 2

(+) Heart Disease (moderate)
(-) Breast Cancer

- You can reduce your risk of heart disease by following the suggestions in "Reducing Heart Disease Risks." The benefits of HRT outweigh the possible increased risk of breast cancer.

- You are currently not at risk for breast cancer; however, just the fact that you are getting older increases your risk. In order to maintain your present status, please follow the "Breast Health" recommendations so you will have a better chance of avoiding this deadly disease.

- If you are not at risk for osteoporosis, or if you are at risk and your BMD is normal, follow the "Bone Health" suggestions to help you continue to have strong bones and prevent hip fractures in the future. You should then repeat your BMD every two to three years.

- If you are at risk for osteoporosis and your BMD indicates osteopenia, following the "Bone Health" suggestions may be sufficient. If you are already on HRT, you may want to consider adding an androgen to your regimen, or using the proper dosage of natural progesterone. Fosamax 5 mg, or Raloxifene 60 mg are also good options. You should then repeat your BMD every two to three years.

- If you are at risk for osteoporosis and your BMD indicates osteoporosis, following the "Bone Health" suggestions may be sufficient. If you are already on HRT, consider adding an androgen. Another option is Fosamax 10 mg, or Calcitonin. Talk with your health-care provider about obtaining bone marker levels before treatment. By repeating the levels in three to six months, you can determine if the treatment is working. You should then repeat your BMD in one to two years.

Please check my website at **www.drcarolle.com** for updated information and research results.

Remember to redo the questionnaires whenever you or a first-degree relative experiences a major health change.

❧ ❧ ❧

SCENARIO #3

(+) Heart Disease (high)
(-) Breast Cancer

- You can reduce your risk of heart disease by following the suggestions in "Reducing Heart Disease Risks." The benefits of HRT definitely outweigh any possible increased risk of breast cancer. Raloxifene could also an option, but more studies are needed to discover whether it decreases the risk of heart disease in the long term.

- You are currently not at risk for breast cancer; however, just the fact that you are getting older increases your risk. In order to maintain your present status, please follow the "Breast Health" recommendations so you will have a better chance of avoiding this deadly disease.

- If you are not at risk for osteoporosis, or if you are at risk and your BMD is normal, follow the "Bone Health" suggestions to help you continue to have strong bones and prevent hip fractures in the future. You should then repeat your BMD every two to three years.

- If you are at risk for osteoporosis and your BMD indicates osteopenia, following the "Bone Health" suggestions may be sufficient. If you are already on HRT, you may want to consider adding an androgen to your regimen, or using the proper dosage of natural progesterone. Fosamax 5 mg, or Raloxifene 60 mg, are also good options. You should then repeat your BMD every two to three years.

- If you are at risk for osteoporosis and your BMD indicates osteoporosis, following the "Bone Health" suggestions may be sufficient. If you are already on HRT, consider adding an androgen. Another option is Fosamax 10 mg, or Calcitonin. Talk with your health-care provider about obtaining bone marker levels before treatment. By repeating the levels in three to six months, you can determine if the treatment is working. You should then repeat your BMD in one to two years.

Please check my website at **www.drcarolle.com** for updated information and research results.

Remember to redo the questionnaires whenever you or a first-degree relative experiences a major health change.

❦ ❦ ❦

Risk Group C:
You are *at risk* for breast cancer only.

Making a Decision about Long-Term HRT
According to Your Personal Risk Level

Below are three scenarios, *only one* of which will match your personal results. Once you find the scenario that matches your results, follow the recommendations, in partnership with your personal health-care provider. Remember, the suggestions given here are only *guidelines* to help you make better decisions for the rest of your life.

SCENARIO #1

(-) Heart Disease
(+) Breast Cancer (average)

- You are currently not at risk for heart disease. Following the "Healthy Lifestyle Changes" suggestions will help you prevent future development of risk. Follow the "Breast Health" recommendations. Whether or not you want to take HRT is a personal decision.

- If you are not at risk for osteoporosis or if you are at risk and your BMD is normal, follow the "Bone Health" suggestions to help you continue to have strong bones and prevent hip fractures in the future. You should then repeat your BMD every two to three years.

- If you are at risk for osteoporosis and your BMD indicates osteopenia, following the "Bone Health" suggestions may be sufficient. Because you are also at risk for breast cancer, Raloxifene 60 mg would be beneficial for your bones as well as conferring you the potential of decreasing your risk of breast cancer, but more studies are needed. Fosamax 5 mg is another option. You should then repeat your BMD every two to three years.

- If you are at risk for osteoporosis and your BMD indicates osteoporosis, following the "Bone Health" suggestions may be sufficient. Another option is HRT. If you are already on HRT, you may want to consider adding an androgen to your regimen, or using the proper dosage of natural progesterone. Another option is Fosamax 10 mg, or Calcitonin. Talk to your health-care provider about obtaining bone marker levels before treatment. By repeating the levels in three to six months, you can determine if the treatment is working. You should then repeat your BMD in one to two years.

Please check my website at **www.drcarolle.com** for updated information and research results.

Remember to redo the questionnaires whenever you or a first-degree relative experiences a major health change.

SCENARIO #2

(-) Heart Disease
(+) Breast Cancer (moderate)

- You are currently not at risk for heart disease. Following the "Healthy Lifestyle Changes" suggestions will help you prevent future development of heart risk. Whether or not you want to take HRT is a personal decision. Follow the "Breast Health" recommendations. Raloxifene could be an appropriate choice in this case because it may decrease your risk of breast cancer, but more studies are needed.

- If you are not at risk for osteoporosis, or if you are at risk and your BMD is normal, follow the "Bone Health" suggestions to help you continue to have strong bones and prevent hip fractures in the future. You should then repeat your BMD every two to three years.

- If you are at risk for osteoporosis and your BMD indicates osteopenia, following the "Bone Health" suggestions may be sufficient. Because you are also at risk for breast cancer, Raloxifene 60 mg would be beneficial for your bones as well as conferring to you the potential of decreasing your risk of breast cancer, but more studies are needed. Fosamax 5 mg is also an option. You should then repeat your BMD every two to three years.

- If you are at risk for osteoporosis and your BMD indicates osteoporosis, following the "Bone Health" suggestions may be sufficient. If you are already on HRT, you may want to consider
  adding an androgen to your regimen, or using the proper dosage
  of natural progesterone. Another option is Fosamax 10 mg, or
  Calcitonin. Talk to your health-care provider about obtaining bone
  marker levels before treatment. By repeating the levels in three to
  six months, you can determine if the treatment is working. You
  should then repeat your BMD in one to two years.

Please check my website at **www.drcarolle.com** for updated information and research results.

Remember to redo the questionnaires whenever you or a first-degree
relative experiences a major health change.

SCENARIO #3

(-) Heart Disease
(+) Breast Cancer (high)

- You are currently not at risk for heart disease. Following the
  "Healthy Lifestyle Changes" suggestions will help you prevent
  future development of heart risk. Follow the "Breast Health" recommendations. Whether or not you want to take HRT is a personal
  decision. Raloxifene could be an option in this case because it may
  decrease your risk of breast cancer, but more studies are needed. If
  there is also a strong family history of both breast cancer and ovarian cancer, genetic testing can be considered. You may also talk to
  your health-care provider about Tamoxifen, prophylactic mastectomy, and oophorectomies (removal of the ovaries).

- If you are not at risk for osteoporosis, or if you are at risk and your
  BMD is normal, follow the "Bone Health" suggestions to help you
  continue to have strong bones and prevent hip fractures in the
  future. You should then repeat your BMD every two to three years.

- If you are at risk for osteoporosis and your BMD indicates osteopenia, following the "Bone Health" suggestions may be sufficient. Because you are also at risk for breast cancer, Raloxifene 60 mg would be beneficial for your bones as well as conferring to you the potential of decreasing your risk of breast cancer. Fosamax 5 mg is another option. You can then repeat your BMD every two to three years.

- If you are at risk for osteoporosis and your BMD indicates osteoporosis, following the "Bone Health" suggestions may be sufficient. Another option is Fosamax 10 mg, or Calcitonin. Talk to your health-care provider about obtaining bone marker levels before treatment. By repeating the levels in three to six months, you can determine if the treatment is working. You should then repeat your BMD in one to two years.

Please check my website at **www.drcarolle.com** for updated information and research results.

Remember to redo the questionnaires whenever you or a first-degree relative experiences a major health change.

❧ ❧ ❧

Risk Group D:
You are at risk for heart disease and breast cancer.

Making a Decision about Long-Term HRT
According to Your Personal Risk Levels

Below are nine scenarios, *only one* of which will match your personal results. To find your personal scenario quickly, use your level of heart disease risk: If it is average, search only Scenario #1 through Scenario #3. If it is moderate, search only Scenario # 4 through Scenario #6. If it is high, search only Scenario #7 through Scenario #9.

Once you find the scenario that matches your results, follow the recommendations in partnership with your personal health-care provider. Remember, the suggestions given here are only *guidelines* to help you make better decisions for the rest of your life.

SCENARIO # 1

(+) Heart Disease (average)
(+) Breast Cancer (average)

- Follow the advice provided in "Reducing Your Risk of Cardiovascular Disease" and "Breast Health." These suggestions may be sufficient. Whether or not you want to take HRT is a personal decision.

- If you are not at risk for osteoporosis, or if you are at risk and your BMD is normal, follow the "Bone Health" suggestions to help you continue to have strong bones and prevent hip fractures in the future. You should then repeat your BMD every two to three years.

- If you are at risk for osteoporosis and your BMD indicates osteopenia, following the "Bone Health" suggestions may be sufficient. Another option is HRT. If you are already on HRT, you may want to consider adding an androgen to your regimen, or using the proper dosage of natural progesterone. Fosamax 5 mg, and Raloxifene 60 mg are also good options. You should then repeat your BMD every two to three years.

- If you are at risk for osteoporosis and your BMD indicates osteoporosis, following the "Bone Health" suggestions may be sufficient. Another option is HRT. If you are already on HRT, you may want to consider adding an androgen to your regimen, or use Fosamax 10 mg, or Calcitonin. Talk to your health-care provider about obtaining bone marker levels before treatment. By repeating the levels in three to six months, you can determine if the treatment is working. You should then repeat your BMD in one to two years.

Please check my website **www.drcarolle.com** for updated information and research results.

Remember to redo the questionnaires whenever you or a first-degree relative experiences a major health change.

❧ ❧ ❧

SCENARIO #2

(+) Heart Disease (average)
(+) Breast Cancer (moderate)

- Follow the advice provided in "Reducing Your Risk of Cardiovascular Disease" and "Breast Health." These suggestions may be sufficient. Raloxifene 60 mg could be an option because of the possibility it decreases breast cancer risk. Repeat your BMD every two to three years. Whether or not you want to take HRT is a personal decision.

- If you are not at risk for osteoporosis, or if you are at risk and your BMD is normal, follow the "Bone Health" suggestions to help you continue to have strong bones and prevent hip fractures in the future. You should then repeat your BMD every two to three years.

- If you are at risk for osteoporosis and your BMD indicates osteopenia, following the "Bone Health" suggestions may be sufficient. Raloxifene 60 mg, and Fosamax 5 mg are also good options. You should then repeat your BMD every two to three years. Whether or not you want to take HRT is a personal decision.

- If you are at risk for osteoporosis and your BMD indicates osteoporosis, following the "Bone Health" suggestions may be sufficient. You may also consider Fosamax 10 mg, or Calcitonin. Talk to your health-care provider about obtaining bone marker levels before treatment. By repeating the levels in three to six months, you can determine if the treatment is working. You should then repeat your BMD in one to two years.

Please check my website at **www.drcarolle.com** for updated information and research results.

Remember to redo the questionnaires whenever you or a first-degree relative experiences a major health change.

❧ ❧ ❧

SCENARIO #3

(+) Heart Disease (average)
(+) Breast Cancer (high)

- Follow the advice provided in "Reducing Your Risk of Cardiovascular Disease" and "Breast Health." These suggestions may be sufficient. Whether or not you want to take HRT is a personal decision. Raloxifene 60 mg could be a good choice in this case, but more studies are needed. If there is also a strong family history of both breast cancer and ovarian cancer, genetic testing should be considered. You should also talk to your health-care provider about Tamoxifen, prophylactic mastectomy, and oophorectomies (removal of the ovaries).

- If you are not at risk for osteoporosis or if you are at risk and your BMD is normal, follow the "Bone Health" suggestions to help you continue to have strong bones and prevent hip fractures in the future. You should then repeat your BMD every two to three years.

- If you are at risk for osteoporosis and your BMD indicates osteopenia, following the "Bone Health" suggestions may be sufficient. Raloxifene 60 mg could be a good choice in this case; Fosamax 5 mg is another option for your bones. You should then repeat your BMD every two to three years.

- If you are at risk for osteoporosis and your BMD indicates osteoporosis, following the "Bone Health" suggestions may be sufficient. Fosamax 10 mg, or Calcitonin are good options. Talk to your health-care provider about obtaining bone marker levels before treatment. By repeating the levels in three to six months, you can determine if the treatment is working. You should then repeat your BMD in one to two years.

Please check my website at **www.drcarolle.com** for updated information and research results.

Remember to redo the questionnaires whenever you or a first-degree relative experiences a major health change.

❧ ❧ ❧

SCENARIO #4

(+) Heart Disease (moderate)
(+) Breast Cancer (average)

- Follow the advice provided in "Reducing Your Risk of Cardiovascular Disease" and "Breast Health." These suggestions may be sufficient. The benefits of HRT may outweigh the risk of breast cancer. Raloxifene could also be an option, but more studies are needed to discover whether it decreases the risk of heart disease and breast cancer in the long term.

- If you are not at risk for osteoporosis, or if you are at risk and your BMD is normal, follow the "Bone Health" suggestions to help you continue to have strong bones and prevent hip fractures in the future. You should then repeat your BMD every two to three years.

- If you are at risk for osteoporosis and your BMD indicates osteopenia, following the "Bone Health" suggestions may be sufficient. Raloxifene could also be an option. If you are already on HRT, you may want to consider adding an androgen to your regimen, or using the proper dosage of natural progesterone. Fosamax 5 mg is also an option. You should then repeat your BMD every two to three years.

- If you are at risk for osteoporosis and your BMD indicates osteoporosis, following the "Bone Health" suggestions may be sufficient. If you are already on HRT, you can consider adding an androgen. Other options are Fosamax 10 mg, or Calcitonin. Talk to your health-care provider about obtaining bone marker levels before treatment. By repeating the levels in three to six months, you can determine if the treatment is working. You should then repeat your BMD in one to two years.

Please check my website at **www.drcarolle.com** for updated information and research results.

Remember to redo the questionnaires whenever you or a first-degree relative experiences a major health change.

❦ ❦ ❦

SCENARIO #5

(+) Heart Disease (moderate)
(+) Breast Cancer (moderate)

- Follow the advice provided in "Reducing Your Risk of Cardio-vascular Disease" and "Breast Health." These suggestions may be sufficient. The benefits of HRT may outweigh the risk of breast cancer.

- If you are not at risk for osteoporosis, or if you are at risk and your BMD is normal, follow the "Bone Health" suggestions to help you continue to have strong bones and prevent hip fractures in the future. You should then repeat your BMD every two to three years.

- If you are at risk for osteoporosis and your BMD indicates osteopenia, following the "Bone Health" suggestions may be sufficient. Raloxifene 60 mg is a good option because of the possibility it decreases the risk of heart disease and breast cancer, and improves your bones. But, remember, more studies are needed regarding the relationship between Raloxifene and heart disease. If you are already on HRT, you may want to consider adding an androgen to your regimen, using the proper dosage of natural progesterone, or Fosamax 5 mg. Repeat your BMD every two to three years.

- If you are at risk for osteoporosis and your BMD indicates osteoporosis, following the "Bone Health" suggestions may be sufficient. You can use any of the following: HRT, HRT plus an androgen, Fosamax 10 mg, or Calcitonin. Talk to your health-care provider about obtaining bone marker levels before treatment. By repeating the levels in three to six months, you can determine if the treatment is working. You should then repeat your BMD in one to two years.

Please check my website at **www.drcarolle.com** for updated information and research results.

Remember to redo the questionnaires whenever you or a first-degree relative experiences a major health change.

❧ ❧ ❧

SCENARIO #6

(+) Heart Disease (moderate)
(+) Breast Cancer (high)

- Follow the advice provided in "Reducing Your Risk of Cardiovascular Disease" and "Breast Health." Whether or not you want to take HRT is a personal decision. Raloxifene 60 mg could be a good choice in this case because of the possibility it decreases the risk of heart disease and breast cancer. If there is also a strong family history of both breast cancer and ovarian cancer, genetic testing should be considered. You should also talk to your health-care provider about Tamoxifen, prophylactic mastectomy, and oophorectomies (removal of the ovaries).

- If you are not at risk for osteoporosis or if you are at risk and your BMD is normal, follow the "Bone Health" suggestions to help you continue to have strong bones and prevent hip fractures in the future. You should then repeat your BMD every two to three years.

- If you are at risk for osteoporosis and your BMD indicates osteopenia, following the "Bone Health" suggestions may be sufficient. Raloxifene 60 mg could be a good choice in this case, especially because of the possibility that it decreases the risk of heart disease and breast cancer, and it is also beneficial for your bones. Repeat your BMD every two to three years.

- If you are at risk for osteoporosis and your BMD indicates osteoporosis, following the "Bone Health" suggestions may be sufficient. For your bones, you can use Fosamax 10 mg, or Calcitonin. Talk to your health-care provider about obtaining bone marker levels before treatment. By repeating the levels in three to six months, you can determine if the treatment is working. You should then repeat your BMD in one to two years.

Please check my website at **www.drcarolle.com** for updated information and research results.

Remember to redo the questionnaires whenever you or a first-degree relative experiences a major health change.

❧ ❧ ❧

SCENARIO #7

(+) Heart Disease (high)
(+) Breast Cancer (average)

- Follow the advice provided in "Reducing Your Risk of Cardiovascular Disease" and "Breast Health." The benefits of HRT definitely outweigh the risk of breast cancer.

- If you are not at risk for osteoporosis, or if you are at risk and your BMD is normal, follow the "Bone Health" suggestions to help you continue to have strong bones and prevent hip fractures in the future. You should then repeat your BMD every two to three years.

- If you are at risk for osteoporosis and your BMD indicates osteopenia, following the "Bone Health" suggestions may be sufficient. Another option is Raloxifene 60 mg, which may decrease the risk of heart disease, as well as being good for your bones; but, more studies are needed. Fosamax 5 mg is also an option. You should then repeat your BMD every two to three years.

- If you are at risk for osteoporosis and your BMD indicates osteoporosis, following the "Bone Health" suggestions may be sufficient. You can also add any of the following: HRT, HRT plus an androgen, Fosamax 10 mg, or Calcitonin. Talk to your health-care provider about obtaining bone marker levels before treatment. By repeating the levels in three to six months, you can determine if the treatment is working. You should then repeat your BMD in one to two years.

Please check my website at **www.drcarolle.com** periodically for updated information and research results.

Remember to redo the questionnaires whenever you or a first-degree relative experiences a major health change.

❧ ❧ ❧

SCENARIO #8

(+) Heart Disease (high)
(+) Breast Cancer (moderate)

- Follow the advice provided in "Reducing Your Risk of Cardiovascular Disease" and "Breast Health." The benefits of HRT may outweigh the risks of breast cancer. Raloxifene is also an option because of the possibility it decreases both heart disease and breast cancer risk, but more studies are needed.

- If you are not at risk for osteoporosis, or if you are at risk and your BMD is normal, follow the "Bone Health" suggestions to help you continue to have strong bones and prevent hip fractures in the future. You should then repeat your BMD every two to three years.

- If you are at risk for osteoporosis and your BMD indicates osteopenia, following the "Bone Health" suggestions may be sufficient. Raloxifene is also an option. If you are already on HRT, you may want to consider adding an androgen to your regimen, or using the proper dosage of natural progesterone. Fosamax 5 mg is another option. You should then repeat your BMD every two to three years.

- If you are at risk for osteoporosis and your BMD indicates osteoporosis, following the "Bone Health" suggestions may be sufficient. You can also add Fosamax 10 mg, or Calcitonin. Talk to your health-care provider about obtaining bone marker levels before treatment. By repeating the levels in three to six months, you can determine if the treatment is working. You should then repeat your BMD in one to two years.

Please check my website at **www.drcarolle.com** for updated information and research results.

Remember to redo the questionnaires whenever you or a first-degree relative experiences a major health change.

❧ ❧ ❧

SCENARIO #9

(+) Heart Disease (high)
(+) Breast Cancer (high)

- Follow the advice provided in "Reducing Your Risk of Cardio-vascular Disease" and "Breast Health." Raloxifene 60 mg could be a good choice in this case because of the possibility it decreases both heart disease and breast cancer. If there is also a strong family history of both breast cancer and ovarian cancer, genetic testing can be considered. You should also talk to your health-care provider about Tamoxifen, prophylactic mastectomy, and oophorectomies (removal of the ovaries). Whether or not you want to take HRT is a personal decision.

- If you are not at risk for osteoporosis, or if you are at risk and your BMD is normal, follow the "Bone Health" suggestions to help you continue to have strong bones and prevent hip fractures in the future. You should then repeat your BMD every two to three years.

- If you are at risk for osteoporosis and your BMD indicates osteopenia, following the "Bone Health" suggestions may be sufficient. Another option is Fosamax 5 mg. You should then repeat your BMD every two to three years.

- If you are at risk for osteoporosis and your BMD indicates osteoporosis, following the "Bone Health" suggestions may be sufficient. You will need to use Fosamax 10 mg, or Calcitonin for your bones. Talk to your health-care provider about obtaining bone marker levels before treatment. By repeating the levels in three to six months, you can determine if the treatment is working. You should then repeat your BMD in one to two years.

Please check my website at **www.drcarolle.com** for updated information and research results.

Remember to redo the questionnaires whenever you or a first-degree relative experiences a major health change.

❦ ❦ ❦

Risk Reduction Recommendations

Here are the recommended references made in each scenario. They include "Healthy Lifestyle Changes," "Reducing Your Risk of Cardiovascular Disease," "Breast Health," and "Bone Health." You should follow what is recommended.

Healthy Lifestyle Changes
- Stress management (chapter 10)
- Healthy nutrition (chapter 11)
- Exercise routine (chapter 14)
- Smoking cessation (chapter 15)
- Use alcohol in moderation (chapter 16)
- Mind-body interventions (chapter 2)
- Keep your weight under control (chapter 13)

Reducing Your Risk of Cardiovascular Disease
- Keep your blood pressure under control (chapter 6)
- Keep diabetes under control (chapter 6)
- Keep your lipid levels under control (chapter 6)
- Keep your weight under control (chapter 13)
- Estrogen (chapter 5)
- Stress management (chapter 10)
- Healthy nutrition, high soy diet, and supplements (chapter 11)
- Exercise regularly (chapter 14)
- Smoking cessation (chapter 15)
- Use alcohol in moderation (chapter 16)
- Mind-body interventions (chapter 2)
- Alternative interventions (chapter 2)
- Aspirin (chapter 6)

Breast Health
- Monthly breast self-exam (chapter 8); report any abnormal findings to your health-care provider
- Yearly breast exam by your health-care provider (chapter 8)
- Regular mammogram: 40 to 50 years old—mammogram every one to two years; 50 years and older—every year (chapter 8)
- Exercise routine (chapter 14)

- Smoking cessation (chapter 15)
- Use alcohol in moderation (chapter 16)
- Keep your weight under control (chapter 13)
- Healthy nutrition, high soy diet, and supplements (chapter 11)

Bone Health

- Stress management (chapter 10)
- Healthy nutrition and high soy diet (chapter 11)
- Exercise routine—with weight-bearing exercise (chapter 14)
- Proper calcium, vitamin D, and mineral intake (chapters 11 and 12)
- Smoking cessation (chapter 15)
- Use alcohol in moderation (chapter 16)
- Use caffeine and soft drinks in moderation (chapter 16)
- Fracture prevention strategies (chapter 7)

Table 20-a
TYPE AND SOURCES OF ESTROGEN

Premarin	Pregnant mare's urine
Estratab	Yam and soy
Ogen	Yam and soy
Ortho-est	Yam and soy
Estrace	Soy
Climara	Soy
Vivelle	Yam and soy
Fem-Patch	Plant source
Dienestroy, Estinyl, Estrovis, Tace	Synthetic materials
Tri-Est	Yam and soy
Estriol cream	Yam and soy
Estring	Yam and soy

Table 20-b

Oral Estrogens	Brand Name	Dosages
Micronized estradiol	Estrace	0.5mg, 1 mg, 2 mg/day
Esterified estrogen	Estratab	0.3 mg, 0.625 mg, 1.25 mg, 2.5 mg/day
	Menest	0.3 mg, 0.625 mg, 1.25 mg, 2.5 mg/day
Quinestrol	Estrovis	0.1 mg, once a week
Estrone sulfate	Ogen	0.625 mg, 1.25 mg, 2.5 mg/day
	Ortho-Est	0.625 mg, 1.25 mg/day
Estropipate	Ortho-Est	0.625 mg 1.25 mg/day
Conjugated equine estrogen	Premarin	0.3 mg, 0.625 mg, 0.9 mg, 1.25 mg, 2.5 mg/day
Estrone 10%, estradiol 10%, estriol 80%	Tri-est (compounded)	1.5 mg bid, 2.5 mg or 5mg /day

Table 20-c

Transdermal Estrogen Patch	Brand Name	Dosages
Estradiol	Climara	0.025 mg, 0.05 mg, 0.075 mg, 0.1 mg, once a week
Estradiol	Estraderm	0.05 mg, 0.1 mg, twice a week
Estradiol	Vivelle	0.0375 mg, 0.05 mg, 0.075 mg, 0.1 mg, twice a week
Estradiol	Alora	0.05 mg, 0.75 mg, 0.1 mg twice a week
Estradiol	FemPatch	0.025 mg, once a week

Table 20-d

Estrogen Vaginal Creams	Brand Name	Dosages
Estradiol	Estrace	0.1 mg in 1 g cream
	Estring silicone ring	2 mg delivered over 90 days
Estropipate	Ogen	1.5 mg in 1 g cream
Dienestrol	Ortho Dienestrol	0.01%
Conjugated estrogen	Premarin	0.625 mg in 1 g cream

Estriol vaginal cream 0.5 mg/gram, (compounded)—¼ tsp at bedtime for one week, then three times weekly thereafter

Estrogen Transdermal Creams	Brand Name	Dosages
Estradiol cream	(Compounded)	0.05 mg/gram, 0.1 mg/gram (⅛ tsp bid)

Table 20-e

Estrogen Injectable	Brand Name	Dosages
Estradiol Valerate	Delestrogen	20–30 mg/month
Estradiol Valerate	(generic)	20–30 mg/month

Table 20-f

Estrogen/Progestin Tablets	Brand Name	Dosages
Conjugated equine estrogen 0.625 mg and Medroxyprogesterone acetate 2.5 mg	Pempro	One tablet/day
Conjugated equine estrogen and Medroxyprogesterone acetate 2.5 mg (MPA included only in 1st two weeks)	Premphase	One tablet/day 0.625 mg
Estradiol 0.5mg and natural micronized progesterone 100 mg	(Compounded)	One tablet/day

Estrogen/Progestin Patch	Brand Name	Dosages
50 mcg estradiol/ 140 mcg norethindrone	CombiPatch	One twice/week
50 mcg estradiol/ 250 mcg norethindrone	CombiPatch	One twice/week

Table 20-g

Estrogen/Androgen Tablets	Brand Name	Dosages
Esterified estrogen 1.25 mg Methyltestosterone 2.5 mg	Estratest	One tablet/day
Esterified estrogen 0.625 mg Methyltestosterone 1.25 mg	Estratest	One tablet/day
Conjugated estrogen 0.625 mg Methyltestosterone 5 mg	Premarin with Methyltestosterone	One tablet/day
Conjugated estrogen 1.25 mg Methyltestosterone 10 mg	Premarin with Methyltestosterone	One tablet/day

Table 20-h

Progesterone	Brand Name	Dosages
Micronized oral progesterone	Prometrium	100 mg
Micronized oral progesterone	(Compounded)	50 mg, 100 mg, 200 mg capsules or suppositories
Natural progesterone cream	(Compounded)	3%, 6%, 10%

Table 20-i

Progestins	Brand Name	Dosages
Medroxyprogesterone acetate	Amen	10 mg
	Curretab	10 mg
	Cycrin	2.5 mg, 10 mg
	Provera	2.5 mg, 10 mg
Norethindrone acetate	Aygestin	5 mg
	Norlutate	5 mg
	Norlutin	5 mg
Mesgesterol acetate	Megace	20 mg, 40 mg
Norgestrel	Ovrette	0.075 mg
Norethindrone	Micronor	0.35 mg
	NorQD	0.35 mg

Table 20-j

Testosterone	Brand Name	Dosages
Testosterone cream	(Compounded)	0.5 mg/gram, 0.5 mg/gram/day
Testosterone capsule	(Compounded)	1.25 mg, 5 mg/twice a day

Conclusion

Every woman is unique and will experience perimenopause and menopause differently. Most women going through natural menopause experience a minimal amount of disturbances during their perimenopausal years and the early menopausal years. For those women who do experience symptoms, the symptoms will alleviate and disappear over a period of time. Until they do, short-term use of HRT, or better yet, alternative remedies, may help.

Some women with risk factors for cardiovascular disease may benefit from the long-term use of HRT, while others with risk factors for breast cancer may not. The decision to choose long-term HRT, alternative treatments, or lifestyle improvements is up to you. Remember that using HRT is not a substitute for a healthy lifestyle. And if you have been using HRT just because years ago you were having symptoms, determine if you need to continue, or stop altogether.

Although the decisions to be made are yours, you will need some help, of course. That is why you have read this book. Therefore, continue to check with your health-care provider, watch television, read magazines and newspapers, and join support or chat groups to keep abreast of new developments.

You should be aware that medical news coverage often focuses on specific, isolated topics, and will not include all the information needed to make individualized choices. If you are a woman of an ethnic minority, you need to know that most research results from clinical studies are skewed because they either do not include women like you, or the numbers of minority women included are usually so small that the findings are not viable. The results, though, do relate to you indirectly and should be considered as you make your choice.

Every woman needs the help of a trusted and knowledgeable health-care provider. However, you should view yourself as a confident person who is able to take charge of your life, and not spend your time worrying about diseases that may occur. By becoming more knowledgeable, you can make better decisions about where to spend your money. With information at hand, you will realize that you have therapy and lifestyle choices, and that these choices can greatly impact your health.

Because your risks will change as you and your relatives age, you should reevaluate these risks every year. Do this on your birthday, during your annual checkup with your health-care provider, or on any memorable date of your choosing, *but do it!*

I trust that you will find the information I have compiled for you in this book helpful. My hope is that I am arming you with the tools to make the right choices for *you*—now and for the rest of your life!

Best of health!
— Dr. Carolle

Afterword

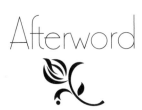

As I walked into the examining room to see my longtime patient, Lisa, I noticed that she was not undressed for a complete physical exam. She was back for another appointment, having had an abnormal Pap smear (and a subsequent one) during her annual visit about ten months prior. Usually, when a patient has an abnormal Pap smear and needs to have it repeated, the time to do her complete annual physical exam is not well defined. I would usually do the complete physical if it is close to the date when the patient would have had her annual exam, as was the case with Lisa.

Handing a gown to Lisa, I told her to completely undress for her physical, and I left the room. When I asked my assistants, Pam and Krista, why Lisa was not prepared, the answer was that, according to Lisa's insurance carrier, she could only have a Pap smear today; an "annual" exam would not be allowed. Lisa would have to come back, at the time her insurance carrier dictated, even though that was less than two months away.

I did not say a word. I went back into the examining room, and before I could explain to Lisa what was going on, I started to cry. It was an awkward moment. Lisa did not know what to do. I guess very few patients had ever seen their doctor crying.

Immense frustration overwhelmed me: It just didn't make sense to do a Pap smear on a patient one visit and then have her return a short time later for a pelvic exam! What about the inconvenience that this ruling by an insurance company caused Lisa, who had to take time from work to come to my office twice? What about the mental trauma that many women, including myself, go through when they have to go to a gynecologist?

I continued to cry, but not just for Lisa. It was also for all my patients who have to deal with so much red tape. It was because we have a medical system that will eventually cause dedicated doctors, nurses, pharmacists, and many other health-care providers to burn out and retire early. I cried for nurses such as my sister, Marise, who has been an intensive-care nurse for the past 14 years; and my sister, Elsie, who has been a psychiatric nurse for the past 12 years, both frustrated with the system but continuing to work because they have bills to pay. I cried for the many times I have heard them and other health-care providers say that they went into medicine when caring for patients was the number-one priority—but that the patient is *not* number one any longer.

I wept for my medical colleagues that I see: sad, overworked, stressed, unhappy, but still dedicated to giving the best care to their patients. I feel for them because I can see that while working in these conditions, eventually their health will suffer. I cried because I know that our society does not realize what is happening, and that should we wake up, we would have lost some of the best and the brightest in medicine—retired at an early age, at the time when their skills are at their peak and so very valuable. I also cried because if Lisa, or anyone, would have asked me what could be done to remedy all this, I would not have had an answer.

I also cried because I realized that as a solo practitioner, I had been fooling myself into believing that I could survive financially while giving the best care to my patients. I was told years ago that doctors in private practice soon would become dinosaurs. I guess my time had come.

I finally told Lisa why I was so upset, and that I would rather quit private practice than continue working in these conditions, where the patient's needs do not come first. I then went ahead with her complete physical exam anyway, as a symbolic gesture.

That night I took a good look at what had been happening to the financial aspect of my practice and realized that for the past two years, I had been experiencing a negative cash flow and had been subsidizing my practice with other income not related to the practice of medicine. I felt so much frustration and anger, and when I realized that the situation could only get worse, I decided that it was time to close my private practice.

Since I had been happy working a morning a week at the Comprehensive Health Center, a clinic that catered to the poor, I called the director, Nora Faine, M.D. I admired her greatly because she had stayed and practiced medicine in the under-served area where she was born and raised. After discussing the decision to close my practice, we agreed that I could come twice a week to her center if I wanted to.

I would also continue with my pro bono work at St. Vincent de Paul Village, and at the Rachel Woman's Center. With my free time, I could do more speaking, writing, return to my belly dancing and painting, learn how to be a storyteller from my friend Alice Smyth-Cooper, and maybe substitute for her at the Nairobi Village at the San Diego Wild Animal Park, telling stories to visitors. I could also make more frequent trips to Haiti to help my people.

When I shared my decision with my husband, Albert, his reply was for me to "do what would make me happy." I also called my relatives and some patients. They all told me that they would support me in any decision I would make: They wanted me to be happy.

So that was it. I would close my private practice. It did not "make me happy" to see patients come in *last* after insurance company rules and the financial "bottom line."

That night, I could not sleep at all. Bleary-eyed and with a heavy heart, I went into the office the next day to find a card from Lisa, the patient whose situation was the "straw that broke *this* camel's back." She wrote that she thought it was a terrible shame when good doctors quit medicine; that I was the first doctor she had ever felt comfortable with, but that she would understand if I quit. It was a long sad day as I mulled over my decision again and again.

It seemed that the universe was trying to tell me something, because the rest of the week my schedule was full of long-term patients whom I have been seeing for years, many staying with me even though they had to pay out of pocket because of insurance obstacles. On the recall list, I saw name after name of patients with whom I had a special bond.

At the end of the week, I received a note in the mail from another patient, thanking me for the extra time I took with her to help her resolve a problem that was not medically related—how as a doctor I help her to heal, and as a woman I empower her. On my bookshelf was *You Can Heal Your Life.* In it, Louise Hay says: "Your mind is a tool you can choose to use any way you wish." Was I allowing my mind to focus on negativity rather than healing?

In between patients, I sat in my office the rest of the day, ignoring the odious insurance paperwork, trying to think with my heart. Finally, a peacefulness came over me. Maybe I felt the presence of my venerable grandfather, or the other healers in my family history, but something made me realize that I could not quit—I am a healer. My relationship with my patients has little to do with money or heartache from the insurance companies, but everything to do with my love of healing, of making a difference in someone's life every day. It truly is in my blood.

What did I learn from this soul searching? I learned that we can find ourselves in situations that make us feel cornered. We then have to take time to sort out our feelings and try to find a solution that will not be detrimental to our health. When I realized that my dealings with insurance companies were killing my soul, and that my practice was, at the moment, a financial burden, I would have been better off financially not going to my office, instead using the time to do other enjoyable things. When I put myself on the brink of making that choice, I was then able to see all the other joys that being in private practice—being my own boss and dealing with my patients in the way I feel is best for them—brings me. Frustration, too, but joy that I can use the gift of healing.

I have to hang on for my patients' sake and for my own. I have to find a way to make it all work. As of this writing, I do not have a solution, but I know things will eventually improve.

❦ ❦ ❦

In addition to questioning my private practice, I also wondered whether I would ever fulfill my dream of having a clinic or a hospital in Haiti. On one visit, I went to Lacou Mirabeau, my grandfather's compound, only to find that the whole place was in shambles. I could not believe my eyes as I gazed upon the abject poverty among my relatives. So, I decided to help the many uncles, aunts, and cousins to rebuild most of their homes, including my grandfather's temple, fence the whole area, and put in a gate that would be closed at night for better security. These people, my own relatives, were very poor, but I hoped that if they had a decent and safer place to stay, it would be easier for them to survive.

I continue to help my relatives financially, and I also support an orphanage outside of Port-au-Prince. But I feel the need to do more.

While I was young in Haiti, it was "foreseen" that someday I would undertake a big project that would benefit many people. When I became a physician in America, I thought that maybe I could become America's first (black) woman surgeon general! But Aiello came, then Elders. And I also could not be the first woman president of the United States because I was not born here. So what would it be, then? Time went by, and the answer didn't come.

Not too long ago, Frantz Lespinasse, a friend who lives in Haiti, asked me why someone like me, who was writing books and giving lectures to empower women here in America, did not do the same in Haiti where it was needed even more? "That is not part of my plan," I told him. "I am already supporting the orphanage and helping my poor relatives."

Then a few days later, I got a phone call from my mother, who had just returned from Haiti. "You have the land to build your school, and your clinic or hospital—whatever you desire!" she told me. One of my cousins, Julie, had unexpectedly inherited over 15 acres of land outside Port-au-Prince. Her father, who had abandoned her as a child, had left everything he owned to her. I called Julie to thank her, and she started to cry while trying to tell me how much it meant to her that I had helped her and my other relatives in Haiti. She said it meant security, hope, pride, life itself, and a lot more. During the embargo, Lacou Mirabeau, with its huge gates, became a safe haven for many people. When Julie saw the huge parcel of land she inherited—so big that she could not see the end of it—she knew that she had to share it with me.

When I hung up the phone, my heart was pounding. The big project I always knew was my destiny will come to fruition in Haiti! Julie's land was giving me that opportunity. Being the founder of a nonprofit organization named "Health Through Communications Foundation," I asked Julie to donate part of her land to the Foundation, and then created a sister foundation in Haiti. I will build a center called "The Center for Learning and Giving." A quote I saw recently summarizes my philosophy about the future center:

"We are each of us angels with only one wing,
and we can only fly by embracing each other."

My dream for this center is to have a primary school, a vocational school for young adults, an outpatient clinic, a nursing school, a convalescent home (Grandma always told me if she had money she would have a place for destitute old women), a minor surgery center, and eventually, a hospital. At the center, all children and young adults who come through the doors will be helped to reach their full potential, and then encouraged to come back to help others. The goal is that by the time of my demise, 200,000 people will have been empowered at the Center for Learning and Giving. I see people from all over the world coming together to make it happen.

In the meantime, I plan to adopt a hospital in Haiti that serves the poor. Maybe it will be the same Albert Schweitzer Hospital that Grandma talked about. I would like to be able to go there several times a year, with a group of health-care providers and ancillary medical personnel, to update preventive care and perform surgeries on a population that is under-served.

I was a little girl from the poorest country in the Western Hemisphere, Haiti, who overcame many obstacles to get to where I am today. Empowering women in five cultures for the past 20 years has been an extremely positive side effect of my "doctoring," but it is just the beginning. . . .

APPENDIX

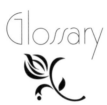

Glossary

A

adrenal glands: small, pyramid-shaped glands situated on top of each kidney that secrete the steroid hormones estrogen, progesterone, and testosterone, as well as various other substances.

amenorrhea: lack of menstrual periods.

amino acid: organic compound of carbon, hydrogen, oxygen, and nitrogen; the "building blocks" of protein.

anovulatory: cessation or suspension of ovulation.

antidepressant: medication or process used to avoid depressive states.

antihypertensive: medication used to lower high blood pressure.

antioxidant: a substance that prevents oxidation or inhibits reactions promoted by oxygen.

arteriosclerosis: used interchangeably with the term *atherosclerosis* to describe a condition affecting the arteries.

atherosclerosis: a variety of conditions where there is thickening, hardening, and/or loss of elasticity of the artery walls, resulting in altered function of tissues and organs

atrophy: withering of an organ that had previously been normal.

B

basal metabolic rate (BMR): temperature of the body at the time of awakening.

benign: noncancerous.

beta carotene: compound in plants that the body converts into vitamin A.

bioflavonoid: constituent of the vitamin C complex.

biopsy: medical procedure taking a small tissue sample in order to confirm a diagnosis.

C

calories: the measure of the energies supplied by the food we eat.

carbohydrates: a chemical compound, found in plants, which include all sugars, starches, and cellulose; a basic source of human energy.

carcinogens: cancer-producing agents.

cardiovascular disease: a general grouping of diseases of the heart and blood vessels.

cell: structural unit of every organism.

cervix: the necklike narrow end of the uterus that opens into the vagina; it stretches to allow a baby to be born.

chlamydia: a bacterial infection of the pelvic organs and urinary tract transmitted by sexual activity.

collagen: a structural protein of the connective tissues.

colorectal: related to the colon (portion of large bowels) and the rectum.

corpus luteum: yellow glandular mass formed by an ovarian follicle after ovulation.

corticosteroid: hormone produced by the adrenal cortex.

cortisone: adrenal hormone that can be harmful to bones; also, a drug that resembles the adrenal hormone.

cyst: a sac of fluid.

cystitis: bladder infection characterized by pain while urinating, a burning sensation, and frequent urination.

D

D&C, or dilation and curettage: medical procedure to scrape away part of the uterine lining (endometrium) to remove abnormal cells.

DNA: deoxyribonucleic acid, the basic molecular subunit of chromosomes.

diabetes: disease caused by failure of the body to produce insulin or to use insulin efficiently, resulting in high levels of sugar in the bloodstream and urine.

diastolic pressure: the period of least pressure in the arterial vascular system.

dysplasia: abnormal development of cells.

E

endocrine glands: glands that secrete hormones into the bloodstream that stimulate or inhibit other body organs.

endometrial biopsy: a small amount of endometrial tissue removed and examined under a microscope.

endometrial hyperplasia: unhealthy buildup of the endometrium due to an imbalance in the levels of estrogen and progesterone.

endometrium: the inner lining of the uterus that builds up and is shed each month.

essential fatty acid: a nutrient that the body can't make but which is essential to good health.

estradiol: a type of estrogen.

estriol: a weaker form of estrogen.

estrogen: female sex hormone found in both women and men, but in a larger proportion in women, primarily responsible for the development and maintenance of female sex characteristics and reproductive functions.

estrone: a weaker form of estrogen.

F

fat: adipose tissue of the body, which serves as an energy reserve.

fluid retention: failure to eliminate fluids from the body because of cardiac, renal, or metabolic disease, or a high level of salt in the body.

follicle: a small sac or cavity composed of cells—for example, the ovarian follicle that produces the ovum.

free radicals: highly reactive molecular fragments, generally harmful to the body.

G

glands: organs that secrete hormones, or other substances that activate or inhibit body functions or that eliminate substances from the body.

gram: unit of mass (weight); about $1/28$ of an ounce.

H

hemoglobin: the iron-containing pigment of the red blood cells.

hemorrhage: heavy bleeding.

hepatitis B: highly contagious type of liver inflammation caused by a viral infection, contracted through contact with infected human blood or with people at high risk for sexually transmitted disease.

herpes: painful and contagious viral inflammatory disease of the skin that causes skin ulcers in the genital and other body areas.

high blood pressure, or **hypertension**: too forceful flow of blood, which may damage the blood vessel walls, leading to heart attack, stroke, or kidney failure.

high-density lipoprotein (HDL): the smallest lipoprotein that removes cholesterol from LDL cells and transports it back to the liver, where cholesterol is broken down into bile acids and excreted into the intestine.

HIV: human immunodeficiency virus, regarded as responsible for the development of AIDS.

hormone: class of chemical substances produced by glands and other body organs that are released into the bloodstream and control various body functions.

hot flash: sudden warmth in the face, neck, or entire body. When it occurs during the night, it is called night sweats.

hyperlipidemia: high cholesterol levels.

hypertension: see **high blood pressure**.

hypothalamus: neural centers of the limbic brain just above the pituitary that control visceral activities, hormone production, water balance, and sleep.

hysterectomy: surgical removal of the uterus.

I

immune: having a high degree of resistance to a disease.

immunization: the process of activating the body's immune response against a specific disease.

impotence: the inability in a male to have an erection or to sustain it until intercourse or ejaculation takes place.

incontinence: inability to control urine retention.

infection: invasion of the body by disease-causing microorganisms, such as viruses and bacteria.

inflammation: reddening and swelling of body tissue as a reaction to infection or cellular injury.

K

kidney: one of a pair of organs located on each side of the lower back that filter waste products from the blood and discard them in urine.

L

lesions: an injury, wound, or a simple infected patch in a skin disease.

libido: sex drive or sexual desire.

lipoproteins: proteins compound of a simple protein and a fat component that carry fats in the blood.

low-density lipoprotein (LDL): particles that are rich in cholesterol.

lumpectomy: removal of a breast cancer without removing surrounding tissue; also see **mastectomy**.

luteinizing hormone (LH): hormone produced by the pituitary gland.

lymphatic system: the vessels and nodes throughout the body that carry the lymph fluid and help to remove toxins from the body.

M

malignant: cancerous.

mammogram: x-ray of the breasts to check for breast cancer in women.

mastectomy, or **radical mastectomy**: surgical removal of a breast cancer and the surrounding tissue; also see **lumpectomy**.

masturbation: self-stimulation of the external sex organs.

menopause: the time of life in which the menstrual period gradually stops and female ovarian hormones decreases.

menorrhagia: excessive bleeding during menstruation.

menstrual cycle: approximately four-week period during which an ovary produces an egg for fertilization, the body sheds an unfertilized egg along with the lining of the uterus (menstruation), and the ovaries again prepare to produce an egg.

menstrual period, or **menstruation**: the monthly flow of blood from the vagina resulting from the uterus shedding its unneeded lining when there is no fertilized egg; also called the **period.**

metabolism: the aggregate of all chemical processes that take place in living organisms resulting in growth, generation of energy, elimination of waste, and other bodily functions as they relate to the distribution of nutrients in the blood after ingestion.

microgram (mcg): one-millionth of a gram.

milligram (mg): a metric unit of weight equal to one-thousandth of a gram.

monosaturated fat: a fat chemically constituted to be capable of absorbing additional hydrogen.

musculoskeletal system: pertaining to the muscles and the skeleton.

myomectomy: removal of a myomatous (muscle-like) tumor of the uterus.

myometrium: muscular wall of the uterus.

N
nanogram: one-billionth of a gram.

nervous system: the extensive, intricate network of structures that activates, coordinates, and controls all the functions of the body.

neurotransmitter: brain chemicals that are involved in carrying messages to and from the brain.

O
occult blood: presence of blood in so small a quantity that it cannot be seen with the unaided eye.

oophorectomy: surgical removal of an ovary.

orgasm: the buildup and release of tension of muscles and nerves during sexual arousal; the climax of sexual excitement.

osteoblast: bone cells that form new bone.

osteoclast: bone cells that reabsorb old bone.

osteopenia: lower-than-normal bone mass.

osteoporosis: thinning of the bones of the body, making fractures more common. After menopause, the risk of osteoporosis usually increases markedly.

ovary: one of two oval-shaped glands located in the female pelvic region that contain eggs and produce the female sex hormones estrogen and progesterone, as well as the male hormone testosterone.

ovulation: the release of an egg from one of the ovaries.

ovum: see **egg**.

oxidation: process of combining with oxygen.

P

Pap smear: taking of a sample of cervical and vaginal cells to detect signs of precancerous conditions.

perimenopausal: the time preceding menopause.

period: see **menstrual period**.

phyto-: denotes relationship to plants.

phytohormones: plant substances that are structurally and functionally similar to human steroids; they exert a very weak effect on the body.

the Pill: birth-control pill that contains the female hormone estrogen, or a combination of estrogen and the female hormone progesterone.

pituitary gland: the body's master gland, located at the base of the brain, which regulates growth and other bodily changes.

placebo: an inactive substance used as if it were an effective dose of a medication.

placebo response: the therapeutic result produced by the belief in a treatment.

plaque: a localized abnormal patch on a body part or surface.

platelet: a round or oval disk found in the blood, important in blood coagulation.

premenopausal: prior to menopause, also called perimenopausal.

progesterone: female sex hormone secreted by the ovaries and adrenal cortex, responsible for the preparation of the uterus for receiving the fertilized egg. Together with estrogen, it helps regulate the monthly period.

progestin: a term usually applied to the synthetic derivatives of progesterone, which differ structurally from progesterone.

progestogen: a term applied to any substance possessing progestational activity; it can refer to progesterone or a progestin.

prolapse: falling of an organ from its normal position.

prophylaxis: steps taken to prevent diseases or their transmission.

pubis, or **pubic area**: frontal bony structure of the pelvis.

Q

qi: the vital life energy which runs through the body (also known as *chi*).

R

radiation: the use of radioactive substances in the diagnosis and treatment of disease.

rectum: lower end of the colon that ends with the anus, or exit point from the body; sometimes a site of sexual excitement and sexual intercourse.

resorption: the loss or dissolving away of a substance.

S

serotonin: substance present in many tissues that stimulates a variety of smooth muscles and nerves and is believed to function as a neurotransmitter.

serum: the watery, noncellular liquid of the blood.

serum cholesterol: cholesterol circulating in the blood.

sexual intercourse: the act in which a man places his erect penis into a woman's vagina; also known as making love, sex, coitus.

sexually transmitted diseases (STDs): infection caused by germs that are spread through sexual contact.

sigmoidoscopy: examination of the intestines through a flexible instrument inserted into the rectum.

stroke: damage to the brain caused by a blood clot or narrowing of a blood vessel so that the blood supply is cut off.

systolic blood pressure: the period of greatest pressure in the arterial vascular system.

T

T lymphocytes (T-cells): a type of white blood cell specializing in the body's defense against viruses and the rejection of foreign tissues.

testes, or **testicles**: two round glands located in the scrotum that produce sperm and the male sex hormone testosterone.

testosterone: male hormone responsible for deepening of the voice and increased hairiness.

thyroid gland: organ at the base of the neck primarily responsible for regulating the rate of metabolism.

tinctures: powdered herbs that are added to a 50-50 solution of alcohol and water.

trichomonas: protozoa that can cause vaginitis.

triglycerides: a combination of glycerol with three or five fatty acids.

tumor: an abnormal mass of tissue that is not inflammatory, arises without obvious cause from cells, and possesses no physiologic function.

U

ultrasound: diagnostic technique that uses sound waves to produce images of internal conditions, such as that of an unborn child, or to diagnose a breast or ovarian cyst.

urethra: tube that leads from the bladder, through which urine is excreted from the body; in the male, it is also the passageway through the penis for the discharge of semen.

uterus: a pear-shaped, hollow, muscular organ located in the female pelvic area, in which the baby develops during pregnancy.

V

vagina: a passageway extending from the uterus to the outside of the body that functions as a female sexual organ and the birth canal.

vaginitis: inflammation of the vagina.

veins: the tubular branching vessels that carry blood from the capillaries toward the heart.

vertebra: any one of the 33 bony segments that make up the spinal column.

X

xeno-: combining form meaning "strange" or "foreign."

Y

yeast: any unicellular, usually oval fungus that reproduces by budding; *candida albicans* is a type of pathogenic yeast.

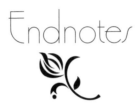

Endnotes

Chapter 2: Alternative Medicine

1. Koff RS. Herbal hepatotoxicity: Revisiting a dangerous alternative. *JAMA.* 1995;273:77-80.
2. Duda RB, Kessel B, Curtin M, Goodman D, Castile M, Eisenberg D, Colditz G, Prouty J, Bookman L. The use of herbal remedies and alternative therapies by breast cancer patients. *Proceedings of Annual Meetings of American Society of Clinical Oncology.* 1995;14-70.
3. Chopra D. *Perfect Health.* New York: Harmony. 1991.
4. Feng LM, Pan HZ, Li WW. Antioxidant action of Panax ginseng. *Chung Hsi I Chieh Ho Tsa Chih.* 1987;7(5):262, 288-290.
5. Hirata ID, Swiersz LM, Zell B, et al. Does dong quai have estrogenic effects in postmenopausal women? A double-blind, placebo-controlled trial. *Fertil Steril.* 1997;68(6):981-986.
6. Foster S. *Garlic.* Botanical Series 311. Austin, TX: American Botanical Council. 1991.
7. Kleijnen J, Knipschild P. Gingko biloba. *Lancet.* 1992;340(8828):1136-1139.
8. Wheatley D. LI 160, an extract of St. John's Wort, versus amitriptyline in mildly to moderately depressed outpatients: a controlled 6 week clinical trial, *Pharmacopsychiatry.* 1997;30(suppl 2):89-90.

Chapter 3: Perimenopause

1. McKinley WM, Brambila DJ, Posner JG. The normal menopausal transition. *Maturitas.* 1992;14:102-115.
2. Francis Hutchins Jr. Uterine Fibroids. Current concepts in Managements. *Female Patient.* 1990;15:29.

Chapter 4: Menopause

1. Nachtigall L, Heilman J. *The Lila Nachtigall Report.* New York: G. P. Putnam. 1977; 165.

2. Margaret L. Contested meanings of the menopause. *Lancet.* 1991;337:1270-1272.
3. Aldercreutz H. Hamalainen E. Gorbach S, Goldin B. Dietary phyto-oestrogens and the menopause in Japan. *Lancet.* 1992;339:1233.
4. Mats H, goran B, Richard L. Does physical exercise influence the frequency of postmenopausal hot flashes? *Acta Obstet Gynecol Scand.* 1990;69:409-412.
5. Freedman R, Woodward S. Behavioral treatment of menopausal hot flushes: Evaluation by ambulatory monitoring. *Am J Obst Gyn.* 1992;167:436-439.
6. Lee J. Natural Progesterone: *The Multiple Roles of a Remarkable Hormone.* Sebastopol, CA:BBL Publishing, 1993;58.
7. Bhatia NN, Bergman A, Karram MM. Effects of estrogen on urethral function in women with urinary incontinence. *Am J Ostet Gynecol.* 1989;160:176-181.

Chapter 5: Hormonal Replacement Therapy

1. Wilson R. *Feminine Forever.* M. Evans and Company, New York. 1966.
2. Grady D, Cebretsadik T, Kerlikowske K, Ernster V, and Petitti D. Hormone replacement therapy and endometrial cancer risk: A meta-analysis. *Obstet Gynecol.* 1995;85(2):304-313.
3. Epstein D: Why women drop out of HRT. *Medical Economics Obstetrics and Gynecology.* January 1998;11.
4. Rodriguez C, Calle EE, Coates RJ, Miracle-McMahill HL, Thun MJ, Health CW. Estrogen replacement therapy and ovarian cancer. *Am J Epidemiol.* 1995;141:828-835.
5. Huley et al. Estrogen plus progestin and CHD. *JAMA.* 1998;280:605-613.
6. Writing Group for the PEPI Trial. "Effects of estrogen or estrogen/progestin regimens on heart disease risk factors in postmenopausal women: The post-menopausal estrogen/progestin interventions (PEPI) trial. *JAMA.* 1995;272(3):199-208.
7. Wingo PA, Layde PM, Lee NC, Rugini G, Ory HW. The risk of breast cancer in postmenopausal women who have used estrogen replacement therapy. *JAMA.* 1987;257:209-215.

Chapter 6: Cardiovascular Disease (CVD) and Women

1. Heart & Stroke A-Z Guide. *American Heart Association.* 1997. URL:http://www.americanheart.org.
2. American Heart Association. *1997 Heart & Stroke Statistical Update.* Dallas, TX: *American Heart Association;* AHA publication 55-0524.
3. Winkleby MA, Kraemer HC, Ahn DK, Varady AN. Ethnic and socioeconomic differences in cardiovascular disease risk factors. *JAMA.* 1998;280(4):356-362.
4. Wenneker MB, Epstein AM. Racial inequalities in the use of procedures for patients with ischemic heart disease in Massachussets. *JAMA.* 1987;261:253-257.
5. Boushey CJ, Beresford SAA, Omenn GS, Motulsky AG. A quantitative assess-ment of plasma homocysteine as a risk factor for vascular disease: probable bene-fits of increasing folic acid intakes. *JAMA.* 1995;274:1049-1057.
6. *The Sixth Report of the Joint National Committee on Detection, Evaluation, and Treatment of High Blood Pressure.* Bethesda, MD. National Heart, Lung, and Blood Institute; 1997. NIH publication 97-4080.

Chapter 7: Osteoporosis

1. Pocock NA, Hopper JL, Yeates MG, Sambrook PN, and Eberl S. Genetic determinants of bone mass in adults: a twin study. *Journal of Clinical Investigations.* 1987;80:706-710.

2. Farmer ME, White LR. Brody JA, Bailey KR. Race and sex differences in hip fracture incidence. *Am J Public Health.* 1984;74:1374-1380.

3. Davies MC, Hall ML, Jacobs HS. Bone mineral loss in young women with amenorrhea. *Br Med J.* 1990;301:790- 793.

4. Fiatarone MA, Marks E, Ryan N, et al. High-density strength training in nonagenarians. *JAMA.* 1990;263:3029- 34.

5. Lindsay R, Tohme JF. Estrogen treatment of patient with established postmenopausal osteoporosis. *Obstet Gynecol.* 1990;76(2):290-295.

6. Ettinger B, Genant HK, Cann CE. Postmenopausal bone loss is prevented by treatment with low-dosage estrogen with calcium. *Ann Intern Med.* 1987;243:1635-1639.

7. Schneider DL, Barrett-Connor EL, Morton DJ. Timing of postmenopausal estrogen for optimal bone mineral density. The Rancho Bernardo Study. *JAMA.* 1997;227:543-7.

8. Christiansen C, Riis BJ. 17 Beta-estradiol and continuous norethisterone: a unique treatment for established osteoporosis in elder women. *J Clin Endocrinol Metab.* 1990;71(4):836-841.

9. Cummings SR, Nevitt MC, Brownwe WS, Stone K, Fox KM, Ensrud KE, Cauley J, Black D, and Vogt TM. Risk factors for hip fracture in white women. *N Engl J Med.* 1995;332:767-773.

10. Eastell R. Treatment of postmenopausal osteoporosis. *N Engl J Med.* 1998;338:736-746.

Chapter 8: Breast Cancer: A Woman's Worst Fear

1. U.S. Department of Health and Human Services. Vital Statistics of the United States. Various years through 1991. Volume II-mortality, Part B. National Center for Health Statistics. 1995; Hyattsville, MD.

2. Lannin et al. Culture, Race, and Breast Cancer Stage. *JAMA.* 1998;279(22)1801-1807.

3. Ambrosone CB, Freudenheim J, Graham S, Narshall JR, Vena JE, Brasure JR, Michalek AM, Laughlin R, Nemoto T, Gillenwater KA, Harrington AM. Shields PG. Cigarette smoking, N-acetyltransferase 2 genetic polymorphisms, and breast cancer risk. *JAMA.* 1996;276:1494-1501.

4. Thune I, Brenn T, Lund E, Gaard M. Physical activity and the risk for breast cancer. *N Engl J Med.* 1997;336:1269-75.

5. Ibid.

6. Bernstein L, Henderson BE, Hanixch R, et al. Physical exercise and reduced risk of breast cancer in young women. *J Natl Cancer Inst.* 1994;86:1403-1408.

7. Ford D, Easton F, Peto J. Estimates of the gene frequency of BRCA1 and its contribution to breast and ovarian cancer incidence. *Am J Human Genet.* 1995;57:1457-1462.

8. Struewing JP, Hartge P, Walcholder S, Baker SM, Berlin M, McAdams M, Timmerman MM, Brody LC, Tucker MA. The risk of cancer associated with specific mutations of BCRA1 and BCRA2 among Ashkenazi Jews. *N Engl J Med.* 1997;336:1401-1408.
9. Schrag D, Kuntz KM, Garber JE, Weeks JC. Decision analysis-Effects of prophylactic mastectomy and oophorectomy on life expectancy among women with BRCA1 or BRCA2 mutations. *N Engl J Med.* 1997;336:1465- 1471.
10. Breast Exam by a Health Care Provider. Reports of the Working Group to review the National Cancer Institute- American Cancer Society Breast Cancer Detection Demonstration Project. *J Natl Cancer Inst.* 1979;62:639-709.
11. Evans JS, Wennberg JE, McNeil BJ. The influence of diagnostic radiography on the incidence of breast cancer and leukemia. *N Engl J Med.* 1986;77:903-909.

Chapter 9: Alzheimer's Disease
1. Evans PH, Klinowski J, Yano E. Cephaloconiosis: A free-radical perspective on the proposed particulate-induced etiopathogenesis of Alzheimer's dementia and related disorders. *Medical Hypotheses.* 1991;34:209-219.
2. Brinton RD, Tran J. Proff HP, et al. 17 beta-estradiol increases the growth and survival of cultured cortical neurons. *Neurochem Res.* 1997;22:1339-1351.
3. Sherwin BB. Estrogenic effects on memory in women. *Ann NY Acad Sck.* 1994;743:230-231.
4. Brenner DE, Kukull WA, Stergachis A, et al. Postmenopausal ERT on risk of Alzheimer's disease-population- based care control study. *Am J Epidemiol.* 1994;140:262-267.
    Paganani-Hill A., Henderson VW. Estrogen replacement therapy and risk of Alzheimer's disease. *Arch Intern Med.* 1996;156:2213-2217.
    Honjo H, Ogino Y, Tnaka K, et al. In vivo effects by estrone sulfate on the central nervous system-senile dementia (Alzheimer's type). *J Steroid Biochem.* 1989;34:521-525.

Chapter 10: Stress and Depression
1. Soloman GF. Emotions, stress, the central nervous system, and immunity. *Annals of the New York Academy of Sciences.* 1969;194(2)335-343.
2. Harvard Mental Health Letter 8 no.7(Jan, 1992).
3. Bartrop RW, et al. Depressed lymphocyte function after bereavement. *Lancet.* 1977;8016(1):834-836.
4. Bahnson CB, Bahnson MB. *Cancer as an Alternative to Psychosis. A Theoretical Model of Somatic and Phychologic Regression.* In Psychosomatic Aspects of Neoplastic Disease, eds. DM Kissen and LL LeShan. Philadelphia: JB Linpincott Company, 1964;184-202.
5. Goleman D. *The Meditative Mind.* Los Angeles, CA: Jeremy P. Tarcher, Inc. 1988;168.
6. Murphy M. *The Future of the Body.* Los Angeles, CA: Jeremy P. Tarcher, Inc. 1992.
7. Stancak A Jr, et al. Observations on respiratory and cardiovascular rhythmicities during yogic high-frequency respiration. *Physiological Research.* 1991;40(3):345-354.

8. D Michaelson, et al. Bone mineral density in women with depression. *J Engl Med.* 1996;335:1176-1181.

9. Wheatley D. LI 160, An extract of St. John's Wort, versus amitriptyline in mildly to moderately depressed outpatients: a controlled six-week clinical trial. *Pharmacopsychiatry.* 1997;30(suppl 2):81-90.

Vorbach EU, Arnoldt KH, Hubner WD. Efficacy and tolerability of St. John's Wort extract LI 160 versus imipramine in patients with severe depression episodes according to ICD-10. *Pharmacopsychiatry.* 1997;30(suppl 2)81-85.

Chapter 11: Implement a Healthy Nutrition Program

1. Stampfer HU, et al. Dietary fat intake and the risk of coronary heart disease in women. *N Engl J Med.* 1997;337:1491-1499.

2. Howe GT, Hirohata T, Hislop TG, et al. Dietary factors and risk of breast cancer: combined analysis of 12 case- control studies. *J Natl Cancer Inst.* 1990;82:561-569.

3. Jeppesen J, et al. Effects of low-fat, high carbohydrate diets on risk factors for ischemic heart disease in postmenopausal women. *Am J Clin Nutr.* 1997;65:1027-33.

4. Dalais FS, Rice GE, Bell FJ et al. *Dietary Soy Supplementation Increases Vaginal Cytology Maturation Index and Bone Mineral Content in Postmenopausal Women. Second International Symposium of the Role of Soy in Preventing and Treating Chronic Disease.* September 15-18, 1996. Brussels, Belgium.

Chapter 12: Calcium and Your Health

1. Devine A, Criddle RA, Dick IM, et al. A longitudinal study of the effect of sodium and calcium intakes on regional density in postmenopausal women. *Am J Clin Nutr.* 1995;62(4):740-745.

2. Nicar MJ, Pak CYC. Calcium Bioavailability from Calcium Carbonate and Calcium Citrate. *Journal of Clinical Endocrinology and Metabolism.* vol. 61 (1985), pp. 391-93.

3. Grossman M, Kirsner J, Gillespie I. Basal and Histalog-Stimulated Gastric Secretion in Control Subjects and Patients with Peptic Ulcer of Gastric Cancer. *Gastroenterolog.* vol. 45 (1963), pp. 15-26.

4. Recker R. Calcium Absorption and Achlorhydria. *N Engl J Med.* vol. 313 (1985), pp. 70-73.

Chapter 13: You and Your Weight

1. Thomas PR, ed. *Weighing the Options: Criteria for Evaluating Weight Management Programs.* Washington, DC: National Academy Press. 1995.

2. Manson JE, Wilett WC, Stampfer MJ, et al. Body weight and mortality among women. *N Engl J Med.* 1995;33:677-685.

3. Pi-Sunyer FX. Medical hazards of obesity. *Ann Intern Med.* 1993;119(7 pt 2):655-660.

4. Manson JE, Colditz Ga, Stampfer MJ, et al. A prospective study of obesity and risk of coronary heart disease in women. *N Engl J Med.* 1990;322:882-889.

5. Carlson KJ, Eisenstat SA, Ziporyn T. *The Harvard Guide to Women's Health.* Cambridge, MA; London, England: *Harvard University Press.* 1996.

Chapter 14: If You're Sedentary, Learn to Exercise
1. Elmer-Dewitt P. *Extra Years for Extra Efforts. Time* 1966:66.
2. Kushi LK, et al, Physical activity and mortality in postmenopausal women *JAMA.* 1997;277:1287-1292.

Chapter 15: If You Smoke, You Must Quit
1. Wenger NK. Hypertension and other cardiovascular risk factors in women. *Am J Hypertens.* 1995;8:94S-99S
2. Jick H, Porter J, Morisson AS. Relation between smoking and age of natural menopause. Report from the Boston Collaborative Drug Surveillance Program, Boston University Medical Center. *Lancet.* 1977;1:1354-1355.
3. Brock K, et al. Smoking and infectious agents and risk of in situ cervical cancer in Sydney, Australia. *Cancer Research.* 1980;49:4925-4928.
4. LaRosa JC. *Coronary Risk Factors in Women.* Presented at the Fourth Chicago Women & Heart Disease Conference. April 25, 1997. Chicago, Il.

Chapter 16: Alcohol, Drugs, and Your Health
1. Smith-Warber SA. Spiegelman D, Yaun SS, et al. Alcohol and breast cancer in women. *JAMA.* 1998;279:535- 540.
    Hernandez-Avila M, et al. Caffeine, moderate alcohol intake, and risk of fracture of the hip and forearm in middle-aged women. *Amer J Clin Nutr.* 1991;54:157-163.

Chapter 17: Sexuality and the Mature Woman
1. Hite, S. *The Hite Report: a Nationwide Study of Female Sexuality.* New York: Dell. 1981; 508.
2. Masters W, Johnson V. *Sex and the Maturing Female. Human Sexual Response.* Boston: Little, Brown and Co. 1966; 177, 238.
3. Bachmann GA. Correlates of sexual desire in postmenopausal women. *Maturitas.* 1985;7(3) (see note 52).
4. Clay VS. Women: *Menopause and Middle Age.* Pittsburgh PA: Know. 1977;92.
5. Coope J. Menopause associated problems. *BMJ.* 1984;289:970-972.
6. Sulak PJ. The perimenopause, a critical time in a woman's life. *Int J Fertil.* 1996;41:85-89.
7. O'Connor D. *How to Make Love to the Same Person for the Rest of Your Life— and Still Love it.* Bantam Books. New York, NY. 1985.

Chapter 19: Take Charge of Your Overall Health
1. Johnson PA, Lee TH, Cook EF, Rouan GW, Goldman L. Effect of race on the presentation and management of patients with acute chest pain. *Ann Intern Med.* 1993;118:593-601.
2. Bergman B, Brismar B. A five-year follow-up study of 117 battered women. *Am J Public Health.* 1991;81:1468- 1469.
3. Varvaro FF. Treatment of the battered woman: effective response of the emergency department. *Am Coll Emerg Physicians.* 1989;11:8-13.

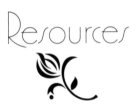

Resources

The following list of resources can be used to access information on a variety of issues. The addresses and telephone numbers listed are for the national headquarters; look in your local yellow pages under "Community Services" for resources closer to your area.

Cancer

- American Cancer Society: (800) ACS-2345
- Cancer Information Service of the National Cancer Institute: (800) 4CANCER
- Susan G. Komen Breast Cancer Foundation: (800) IM-AWARE
- Women Health Initiative Research Centers: For one near you, call (800) 54WOMEN
- Y-ME National Organization for Breast Cancer Information: (800) 221-2141

Compounding Pharmacies

To locate a compounding pharmacy near you, contact the International Academy of Compound Pharmacies (IACP) • (800) 927-4227 • fax (713) 495-0620 • www.iacp.com/iacp or the Professional Compounding Centers of America, Inc. (PCCA) at (800) 331-2498 • fax 800-874-5760 • www.compassnet.com/pcca/

- Jerry Greene, chief compounding pharmacist, University Compounding Pharmacy • (800) 985-8065 • www.ucprx.com

Fitness

- American Council on Exercise, P.O. Box 910449, San Diego, CA 92121

- 800-529-8227 • www.acefitness.org

- Becky Cortez, ACE-certified personal trainer/fitness expert for ABC. Fitness for Health • (888) 333-5348

General Health

- National Women's Health Network, 514 10th Street NW, Suite 400, Washington, DC 20004 • (202) 347-1140 • (202) 628-7814 (publications)

- For information about soy foods, write to the Soy Foods Association of America, 1 Sutter St., Suite 300, San Francisco, CA 94104 (include a business-size SASE)

Heart

- American Heart Association, National Center, 7272 Greenville Ave., Dallas, TX 75231 • 800- AHA-USAI • www.amhrt.org

Hypnosis

To find an experienced hypnotist, call the Institute for Clinical Hypnosis in Great Neck, New York • (516) 482-1220

Menopause

- The North American Menopause Society, P.O Box 94527, Cleveland, OH 44101-4527 • www.menopause.org

Mental Health

- National Institute of Mental Health, 5600 Fishers Lane, Room 7C-02, Rockville, MD 20857- 8030 • 301-443-4513 • 800-969-6642 • www.nimh.nih.gov

Osteoporosis

- National Osteoporosis Foundation, Dept. MQ., P.O. Box 96616, Washington, DC 20077-7456 • (800) 223-9994

Smoking Cessation

- The American Cancer Society, National Headquarters,1599 Clifton Road NE, Atlanta, GA 30329 • 800-ACS-2345 • www.cancer.org

San Diego-Area Resources

Since I consider myself a native San Diegan, I am providing some resources specifically for my friends in Southern California:

- Steve Haynes, M.A., physical therapist/personal trainer • (619) 583-4955

- The Brighter Side, a Boutique for Women with Cancer, 439 So. Cedros Ave., Solana Beach, CA 92075

- Belly Dancing—Magical Motion with Althea and Friends. Magical Motion Enterprises, 12228 Venice Blvd., Ste. 402, Los Angeles, CA 90066 • (310) 301-0045 • atea@anet.net

- Karen Gless, Ph.D., marriage, family, and child counselor specializing in sex therapy, San Diego, CA • (619) 565-1069 www.Hypno-Tapes.com/hypnosis

- Lisa Smith, psychotherapist, Encinitas, CA 92024 • (760) 943-1567

- Sabrina Cox, foot and hand reflexology, San Diego, CA (619) 590-6929

- Adela C. Albrektsen, L.Ac, licensed acupuncturist and Chinese herbalist, San Diego, CA • (619) 960-4649 (voice mail pager)

- Marie Kastner, licensed acupuncturist and herbalist • (619) 220-0878

- Susan Foley, Ph.D., O.M.D., L.Ac., Acupuncture, San Diego, CA
  (619) 275-0550

- Gloria T. Sigafoos, P.T., O.C.S., Biofeedback for Bladder Incontinence,
  San Diego, CA • (619) 452-0282

- Doreen Borsett, D.C., chiropractor, San Diego, CA • (619) 576-6900

- Louis A. Gregory, D.C., chiropractor, San Diego, CA • (619) 454-6788

- Linda Meyers, whole foods nutritional information • (800) 581-0935

- Sandra Schrift, career coach to professional speakers, San Diego, CA
  (619) 460-7866 • sschrift!grossmont.k12.ca.us

Recommended Reading

Alternative Medicine, by the Burton Goldberg Group

Basket of Blessings, by Karen O'Connor

Body and Soul: The Black Women's Guide to Physical Health and Emotional Well-Being. A National Black Women's Health Project Book, Linda Villarosa, editor

Complete Guide to Women's Health, by the American Medical Association

Dr. Susan Love's Hormone Book, by Susan M. Love, M.D., with Karen Lindsey

Empowering Women: Every Woman's Guide to Successful Living, by Louise L. Hay

Fantastic Water Workouts, by MaryBeth Pappas Gaines

For Yourself: The Fulfillment of Female Sexuality, by Lonnie Garfield Barbach

Heal Your Body A-Z, by Louise L. Hay

Herbs for Health and Healing, by Kathi Keville, with Peter Korn

The Menopause Industry, by Sandra Coney

Menopause Without Medicine, by Linda Ojeda, Ph.D.

Overcoming Addiction Without a Twelve Step Conviction, by Oliver Rhodes
To order, call (619) 491-0559 • fax (619) 293-3166 • E-mail: bcoolu@aol.com

Peace Train to Beijing and Beyond, by Beth Glick-Rieman

Preventing and Reversing Osteoporosis, by Alan R. Gaby, M.D.

Relaxation and Breathing Techniques, by Herbert Benson M.D.

The Simple Soybean and Your Health, by Mark and Virginia Messina

Timeless Healing, by Herbert Benson, M.D.

The Western Guide to Feng Shui: Creating Balance, Harmony, and Prosperity in Your Environment, by Terah Kathryn Collins

Women's Bodies, Women Wisdom, by Christiane Northrup, M.D.

You Can Heal Your Life, by Louise L. Hay

About the Author

Carolle Jean-Murat, M.D., F.A.C.O.G., was born into a family of traditional healers. From them she learned to care deeply and listen intently to patients, to understand that health and medicine have spiritual and emotional components, and to heal the *whole person*—not just symptoms.

Dr. Carolle is a board-certified obstetrician and gynecologist, and a Fellow of the American College of Obstetricians and Gynecologists. She has had a private practice in San Diego, California, since 1982. Fluent in five languages, she provides medical care and preventive health education to women of diverse backgrounds. For over a decade, she has been providing free medical care to under-served women through Catholic Charities and St. Vincent de Paul Village.

Dr. Carolle is an Assistant Clinical Professor at the University of California at San Diego (UCSD) School of Medicine, Dept. of Reproductive Endocrinology. She is also a clinical mentor for under-served students at San Diego State University. She is a motivational speaker who brings her message of *self-empowerment* to women through lectures, TV and radio appearances, a Spanish-language newspaper column, articles, and audiocassettes.

Dr. Carolle is the author of an award-winning book, *Staying Healthy: 10 Easy Steps for Women,* available in both English and Spanish; and *Natural Pregnancy A–Z.*

YOU MAY CONTACT DR CAROLLE:

By mail:	5555 Reservoir Drive, Suite 310
	San Diego, CA 92120
By phone:	(619) 583-5061
By fax:	(619) 583-2114
By e-mail:	info@drcarolle.com
Through her website:	www.drcarolle.com

Notes

Notes

Notes

Notes

Notes

Notes

Notes

Notes

Notes

Notes